Ageing Safely in the Home of YOUR Choice

Ideas and Tips to Customize your Home
into a Senior-Friendly Environment

JEAN-FRANÇOIS PINSONNAULT

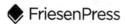

FriesenPress

One Printers Way
Altona, MB R0G 0B0
Canada

www.friesenpress.com

Copyright © 2022 by Jean-François Pinsonnault
First Edition — 2022

The author of this book disclaims liability for any loss or damage suffered by any person or organization as a result of the information or content in this book. The ideas, suggestions, and tips contained herein are based on the author's own experience and circumstances as a family caregiver and are for educational purposes only. They represent the family and his personal life situations and challenges. Please consider that you, the reader, have unique conditions and concerns of your own and my experiences may not have beneficial outcomes for you. Consult an Occupational Therapist for further guidance.

ISBN
978-1-03-912888-0 (Paperback)
978-1-03-912890-3 (eBook)

1. *Self-Help, Aging*

Distributed to the trade by The Ingram Book Company

Table of Contents

Acknowledgements

Thank you, thank you, thank you to all the spouses, sons, sons-in-law, nephews, other extended male family members, and friends who have stepped up and have been and continue to be active family caregivers—a wholehearted thank you.

I believe that many males silently want to be more involved in caring for their parents and other family elders when such support and involvement is required. However, because of centuries-old messaging, unfortunate past or broken relationships, or deep-seated inner anxieties and fears, many men shy away from the beautiful opportunity for adult children and parents to rediscover and appreciate each other. All I can say is, you are not alone. It is, sadly, a frequent reaction. But you've got this. Ignore these old-fashioned views, and step up. You will not regret it.

Most importantly, I am profoundly grateful and appreciative to the spouses, daughters, daughters-in-law, nieces, extended female family members, and friends who, for centuries, have been the ones who cared for their elders—a heartfelt thank you. You are all our heroes. Do not let up. As your children grow up, boys and girls, show them the importance of respect, kindness, and the responsibility of caring for others in need. As parents, it starts with you. As you well know, the responsibility of caregiving is very demanding. Enlist others to help and support you. Please do take the time to care for yourself, too. Find opportunities to take small breaks and time off to re-energize.

Parents, sadly, often do not ask for help. Regrettably, this too, is a persistent reaction. Keeping one's independence and control is paramount for seniors. They do not want to be an imposition or a bother in your life. Look for clues or signs of unusual actions or behaviours, which are often indicators that it's not like it was when you were growing up. They need you!

Always be gentle and patient in raising your observations and concerns. Find the right moment. In front of other family members and friends is never the opportune time to spring the subject on your parents or grandparents. Remember, it is challenging for seniors to ask for help. Processing such a request of their children is frequently interpreted as the beginning of the end. Instead, find ways to support them in their desires of remaining in their home for as long as possible.

Jean-François Pinsonnault

Male and female family members are, and I can appreciate this, very busy and may not have the time or will to care for their parents. Nonetheless, I can clearly say that, as a son with an active career, though challenging, requiring organization, and sometimes overwhelming, I found the time and the resources to permit me to be the principal caregiver for my mother for over a decade. I can unequivocally state that my involvement was instrumental in my mom living many years beyond what would have probably transpired had I accepted placing my mother in a long-term care facility.

I dedicate this book to seniors who, while living in their home, might be experiencing some challenges, and to everyone who is a dedicated caregiver to the current and future elders, who appreciate their family's support. I only hope you will find these ideas, suggestions, and tips helpful during your life journey.

*No matter what you've done for yourself or humanity, if you can't look back on having given love and attention to your own family, **what have you really accomplished**?*
— Lee Iacocca

INTRODUCTION

Elders are the backbone of our civilization. For generations, they have toiled to give their children and families the best lives they could, often making personal sacrifices for their family's betterment. Great-grandparents and grandparents, in many instances, participated in our upbringing with love and tenderness. Previous generations experienced wars, depression, and unemployment. Dishearteningly, a debilitating pandemic has decimated many seniors for over a year now. Our elders need us more than ever.

Over 90 percent of seniors live an active lifestyle in their homes or some form of retirement communities. The National Institute on Ageing/TELUS Health Survey[1] conducted in July 2020 revealed that almost 100 percent of Canadian seniors aged sixty-five and up would do everything in their power to remain in the house of their choice for as long as they possibly can.

This book highlights quickly and often easily made actions, adjustments, and changes, several at no or little cost, to increase their wellness and transform their environment into a safe and comfortable senior-friendly home, where they can remain for years to come. Many of these ideas are based on my own experience and circumstances as a family caregiver to my mother for fourteen years. They represent the situations and challenges I experienced with my mother, my personal life, and conversations I have had the honour of having with hundreds of seniors. Every so often, I will share some of these heart-warming stories, in a gray shaded box on the page.

Please consider that you, the reader, have unique conditions, challenges, and concerns of your own, and my experiences may not have the same beneficial outcomes for you. Nevertheless, I hope that these pages will start personal reflection, leading to valuable and fruitful conversations with family members.

Jean-François Pinsonnault

PART 1
Why Me? Why Now?

I am a son who was the principal caregiver for my mother for fourteen years. At that time, little information was available. My learning curve was steep. Through trial and error, I learned ways to make a senior's life more comfortable without putting them in a long-term care facility or retirement home. Mother's challenges were numerous. She had several limitations: mobility challenges due to lesions on her legs and limited vision, a propensity for strokes, and, later discovered, type 2 diabetes.

I resisted the insistence to institutionalize my mother after she spent months in the hospital. Instead, as per Mom's wishes, plus the fact that I could safely address her medical challenges, I organized everything for her return to the family farmhouse, with my support, the help of a live-in companion, and the few community services of the day.

Midway through the COVID-19 pandemic, listening like many to the evolution and impact of the virus, I noted several doctors expressed their frustration at the number of seniors residing in long-term care facilities. From their perspective, it was possible that up to 30 percent of seniors, with proper guidance and information, would have been better off staying in their home, supported by the appropriate home care services.

Unfortunately, most health system's resources for the elderly are directed to hospitals and long-term care with minimal support, if any, to home care. The seemingly total disregard for the elderly by so many governments triggered my anger, which is extremely rare for people who know me. At that moment, I felt I had to do something tangible.

As I had personally experienced home caregiving for my mother, I learned how to adjust her living environment into a senior-friendly home. On many occasions before the pandemic, I shared with others many of the ideas, suggestions, and tips that could be helpful to seniors. I also researched and pulled all the best practices from different countries into a book for seniors and their families who wish to remain living in their current home or any other type of housing arrangement they choose for as long as possible.

CHAPTER 1

My Caregiving Journey

In the early 1980s, two years after my father passed away from a heart attack in his sleep, my mother suffered a debilitating stroke. Subsequently she had a lengthy stay at the Montreal Neurological Institute-Hospital, about an hour's drive from the family home. After several months of challenging recovery, her doctors informed us they had done what they could and strongly suggested she go into a nursing home to continue her recovery. When my older siblings agreed with the doctor's suggestion, I was appalled and shocked. I could not have fathomed that my sisters and brothers were ready to give up so quickly on Mother. My reaction was swift: No!

As the youngest child of five, I had been ill with rheumatic fever during my formative years, and my mother cared for me for nearly two years until I recovered and could go back to school. During this time, we established a solid bond. As I matured, I often reflected on the time my mother had cared for me, and I decided that should my parents ever need me during their senior years, I would be there for them.

Based on previous conversations with my mother on the subject, I knew she preferred to go back to her own home with additional support and adjustments, like the majority of seniors today. So I set out a plan and made the appropriate arrangements. Though challenging, a live-in companion was eventually found and hired. Unfortunately, it was not easy to find the right person. It took a couple of attempts to find the gem that would care for my mother for nearly ten years.

Relatively straightforward adjustments and changes were made to various rooms in her house to increase her comfort, safety, and wellness. For example, Moms bedroom was moved to the main floor, near the washroom, eliminating the need to use the long stairway, which was quite challenging because of her frailness. In addition, for ten years, I travelled to the farm and filled in for my mother's companion every other weekend to give her some time off and a couple of weeks for summer vacation and popular holidays.

I prepared meals, engaged in conversation about our lives since our last encounter, reminisced, and explored the future. Once Mother's strength had improved, we sometimes went shopping and stopped in to see some of her friends who lived in the village nearby. I often suggested that whenever she was ready, she was welcome to come and live with me. Her response was always the same: "One day, maybe, but I am not ready now."

One spring day, after ten years of being her weekend, birthday, holiday, and on-call caregiver, she phoned me between visits and asked, "Is the offer still good?"

There was a short pause between her question and my response, which at the time seemed like an eternity. What would this mean for her and my bohemian lifestyle? Would I be able to care for her as she had for me so many years prior? Where would we live? When was my mother expecting to arrive? What if her condition got worse? What impact would this new arrangement have on my career? Was I up to the challenge? I was now living about almost three hours away in a neighbouring province, could I find the appropriate area to live-in that had the support services mother needed?

"Yes, of course it is," was my response. Though our impromptu conversation was unexpected, given that I had asked my mother to move in with me so often, we both felt ecstatic and happy about the future that lay ahead of us. We both looked forward to the next months of planning and organization for the move.

We continued our conversation, during which she answered several of my questions. Mother wanted to spend her last summer on the farm. It would take nearly a year to understand her rational for that timeline. Late October became the target arrival date. When it came time to determine how we would inform the rest of the family, which I knew would not be easy, we agreed to do it on Mother's Day, about a month away. These few weeks would give me time to organize everything. We had a strategy.

Throughout the years, all the children attempted to make their way to the farm to celebrate birthdays and special holidays, including some vacation time with our parents. During the years after the passing of my father and Mother's illness, I took over the organization of these events. I would usually arrive a few days before to organize and prepare all the food. Some years, when pressed for time, I would reach out and ask each family to bring a dish to complement the menu.

As the youngest of the family, I did stay the longest with my parents on the farm. At a very early age, I would watch my mother prepare meals and ask lots of questions. So I knew all or at least most of her culinary secrets. Over the years, I discovered and explored different cooking styles and cultures in a small café I co-owned and operated with two associates.

I spent the next several weeks planning how I would go about telling the family, exploring options with my mother during my regular visits.

CHAPTER 2

Matching Mother's Needs
to a Future Home

I researched all the areas best suited for seniors to live comfortably. There were towns in various parts of the country. However, I did not want to be too far from the rest of the family. It so happened that Ottawa had numerous community services that we could call upon for support, and my older sister and husband and their two sons lived in the area, and other family members would be about a two-hour drive away.

Though I had declined a position in Ottawa less than three months earlier, I contacted the manager who had originally suggested I apply for the job. To my surprise, the organization had chosen none of the applicants. After a brief conversation about why I was now interested, she encouraged me to apply again. Four months later, I started working in Ottawa, living in my sister's basement in the west end of the city, until I found a suitable place to purchase for my mother and me.

I spent all my free time driving around the surrounding area to try and locate a suitable place to live. One challenge I quickly experienced was the traffic congestion both going to and coming from work. It was a horrendous nightmare, rarely taking less than ninety minutes. So I decided that east of the city would be the best commuting option. The early morning and afternoon sun would always be behind me, and based on feedback from work colleagues, the traffic density was far less.

Mother had lived in a rural setting for a very long time, so I was looking for a small bungalow with everything she needed on the main floor and a finished basement for my quarters. The focus was on finding a house that met our needs and comfort, located in a quiet area with trees, a garden, a place to grow flowers, and hopefully some space for a small vegetable garden.

My first realtor did not pan out, as he kept bringing me to visit houses that had all the criteria I had explicitly said I did not want: steps to a sunken living room, a step between the kitchen and the dining room, and a baseboard heating system—which is not ideal for maintaining a constant temperature for a senior's comfort.

There was no space to sit outside, no patio, and no trees or quiet area for a garden. Finally, after nearly five weeks of showing the same type of properties with the same inadequacies and out of frustration, I cancelled the relationship and took a few days to regroup.

One day after work, I stopped at the store to purchase a few things at a grocery store that my sister had forgotten to pick up. Relatively new to the city, I stopped at the first store I saw. After looking up and down a few aisles, I found the items she wanted. As I exited, a display of magazines caught my eye. It was all about houses for sale and their general location around the city. These weekly magazines became my source of information.

After a few weeks and several grocery store and shopping mall trips, I narrowed my search to three possibilities situated in the east or southeast of the city. The descriptions read well, and the pricing was within my range. In the meantime, one of my work colleagues suggested a realtor they had used a year before. I followed up, and the phone conversation went surprisingly well. We agreed to meet the next day during lunch. We spent the first fifteen or so minutes getting to know each other. In response to his inquiry, I shared the criteria of what I was seeking and in what general location. I then showed him the three properties I had identified. His reaction was immediate. He would call the listing agents and make arrangements for a visit the following weekend.

He picked me up on Saturday morning, informing me that he had found a fourth possible property that met my wish list. We visited all four, and though they met my basic needs, the first one really caught my eye: an acre lot; a bungalow with few steps to enter; the main floor with everything Mother would appreciate including a fireplace, which she had always wanted; a large patio accessible from the dining room, facing a forest that was part of the region's greenbelt; and lots of privacy. Later that afternoon, I made an offer, and barring a few basic expected requirements, everything went well. Within a few days, the purchase was complete.

Mother had developed sores on her legs over the years that required frequent fresh bandages, and her eyesight had diminished significantly. Declared legally blind several years prior, she had tunnel vision. Nevertheless, she could get around with care. Everything on the main floor was the perfect setup for us. And on top of it all, driving to work was about a half-hour trip. The proximity of all the support services and shopping options Mother would require was a big plus.

The following four years would open up countless events and situations, most of which would be delightful, heartening, and simply memorable. Others, however, would fall into the category of surprising, challenging, and in the moment, quite overwhelming. Mother passed nearly four years later due to complications from a terrible stroke. I grieved her passing for several years, trying to write various aspects of our journey; however, I struggled to write something meaningful as the grief and emotions overwhelmed me.

I retired in December 2011, and for the first three months, I pondered what I was going to do with my future career. Then, a dear friend helped me through an assessment tool called the "Passion Test," which narrows one's future interests and goals. Lo and behold, the top goal was to write and publish a memoir about our journey, the second one, linked to the first, was to influence boys and sons to take a more active role in caring for their parents, and the third was to continue teaching, which I still am involved with today.

If so inclined, you can read all about it in my published work, *Lasting Touch – A Mother and Son's Journey of Joy, Challenges, Sadness, and Discovery*, by Jean-François Pinsonnault.

PART 2
Ageing Challenge

"Ageing is a triumph of development. Increasing longevity is one of humanity's greatest achievements. People live longer because of improved nutrition, sanitation, medical advances, health care, education, and economic well-being…

…A report from the United Nations Population Fund identifies gaps and provides recommendations for the way forward to ensure a society for all ages in which both young and old are given the opportunity to contribute to development and share in its benefits. A unique feature of the report is a focus on the voices of older persons themselves, captured through consultations with older men and women around the world."[2]

As a point of reference, both genders' average life expectancy in Canada in early 1800 was just below forty years. However, by early 1900, it had slightly increased to around fifty years. In 2021, the life expectancy for both genders averages eighty-three years.[3]

Throughout these 200-plus years, the low life expectancy increased very slowly because of pneumonia, tuberculosis, enteritis, and influenza, which impacted 40 percent of children under five years old. Fortunately, the twentieth century brought medical discoveries such as antibiotics and vaccines.

Though WWI (1914–18), the devastating influenza pandemic (aka Spanish flu; 1918–19), and WWII (1939–45) created a kind of plateauing effect on life expectancy, it also created a positive impact because of the discovery and application of beneficial medical and health care advancements.

CHAPTER 3

Canada's Health Systems

Canada's health care system dates back to the mid-1950s when life expectancy was around the mid-sixties. Regrettably, it is based on doctors and acute care[4] in hospitals and not on seniors' needs with a longer life expectancy and complex chronic diseases.[5] Canada's life expectancy has significantly increased compared to the out-dated perspective and focus of that era. Technological advances in medicine have considerably impacted longevity. Sadly, the transitioning to supported home care services has not.

Furthermore, in a recent online survey conducted between November 27 and December 1, 2020, most Canadians aged sixty-five years and older will do everything they can to avoid moving into a long-term care (LTC) home as they get older, an increase of around 10 to 13 percent from before the pandemic.[6]

According to health policy advocates such as the National Institute on Ageing and the Ontario Community Support Association, a higher level and quality of home care should be widely available to seniors.

"The benefit of increased homecare investment in Canada is getting long-overdue attention. Now that COVID-19 has torn through long-term care homes, killing thousands of residents and exposing fatal weaknesses in the system," said Dr. Samir Sinha, head of geriatrics at Mount Sinai and University Health Network hospitals in Toronto.[7]

People of different generations have witnessed parents, grandparents, and other extended family members who, unprepared for ageing, endured physical, emotional, and psychological hardship and challenges as they aged. These personal life experiences have brought about a higher level of awareness and focus on what their future might hold. Sadly, such a future perspective was not common in the twentieth century and indeed is still not sufficiently predominant in today's environment, as described and observed in a recent documentary called *Fast Forward*. [8]

My mother's own experiences with her parents and family members were instrumental in ensuring she would do everything possible to maintain her independence for as long as possible. Luckily, mainly because my parents paid close attention to an influential uncle and the many hardships of the early twentieth century, they still managed to plan a comfortable life for their golden years. Unfortunately, my father did not benefit very long from his planning, as he passed away in his early seventies of a heart attack. Nonetheless, my mother could support herself and have a live-in companion care for her because of this foresight, as there was little support available for the elderly from the day's health care system.

The Canadian Institute of Health Information (CIHI) analyzed the health status of people admitted to long-term care facilities in Canada. It concluded that **one in nine new long-term care residents potentially could have been cared for at home** with ongoing home care support availability.[9]

During the nearly four years my mother lived with me, the province provided various home care services that significantly enhanced Mom's quality of life: fifteen hours per week for a personal support worker, weekdays while I was at work. For additional support, I contracted an extra two hours per day for a total of twenty-five hours weekly. Furthermore, I organized and adjusted our home to a senior-friendly environment to make Mom's life easier and more comfortable, like I had done in her home following her hospital stay. Among the services provided were regular visits by a nurse from the Victorian Order of Nurses (VON), training on how to change bandages on her legs, home delivery of medical supplies, monthly visits by a social worker to chat with my mother about her well-being, etc.

As it was then and is still prevalent today, it is a sad fact that many seniors end up in long-term care facilities for several reasons:

- **Poor communication:** The option of going back to their home is often not discussed by many medical professionals, as I experienced with Mother's doctors. The narrative about ageing remains stuck in the past, as does the prejudice facilitated by widespread ageism. It seems that this is the last "ism" still unaddressed in society. It's still acceptable and tends to dominate conversations and discourses among politicians, medical professionals, and sadly, younger populations.

- **Lack of innovative thinking:** I think institution-alization has become the go-to answer for many medical professionals and governments, with little consideration for organized and available pertinent and quality home care services.

- **Insufficient funding:** The health care system does not genuinely consider or prioritize the benefits of consistent and appropriate home care services. The result is inadequate funding for adequate and quality home care services. Other countries have shown reductions in health costs when using home care instead of hospitals and long-term care institutions.

Based on 2015 figures,[10] Canada spends 87 percent of its public investments in health care in long-term care versus 13 percent on home and community-based care, which is well below other member countries of the Organisation for Economic Co-operation and Development (OECD). For instance, the United Kingdom, Belgium, Norway, and Denmark spend between 40 and 60 percent on home and community-based care. Though some improvements have occurred, Canada still has a long way to go.

CHAPTER 4

Impact of the Pandemic

The COVID-19 pandemic has, without any doubt, been horrific for seniors in long-term care (at least three times the rate of outbreaks compared to retirement homes and seven times the rate of outbreaks in Ontario hospitals) and retirement facilities. The lack of preparedness by most of the world is not surprising.

When tragic, destructive, and often fatal events occur somewhere in the world, strange and inexplicable reactions by people and governments seem to occur. For some, it is something happening to somebody else far away, so we disregard it. Others have become jaded and do not care, while others are distracted by trivial issues and do not pay attention to anything except their closed world.

Since 1970, several dozen infectious diseases have emerged from human interaction with animals and nature, including SARS, H1N1 (swine flu), MERS, avian flu (H7N9), Ebola, Zika, and now COVID-19, to name but a few. For fifteen years, the World Health Organization warned that infectious diseases were emerging at a rate not seen before. Yet after each pandemic, governments failed to develop a strategy for the future or did not act on it if they did produce one. Most past and present governments ignored the warnings from the health and scientific communities and senior health-related advocacy groups.

The fundamental principle of the Canadian health care system is equal medical access for all. However, the pandemic events clearly show that when it comes to ageing, vulnerable, and racialized populations, these groups fall through its wide cracks. As it pertains to the growing number of seniors, the old standards and the current health care models no longer address and meet its citizens' needs.

Though various advocacy groups and seniors themselves raised issues, challenges, and pitfalls for countless years, reality has shown that multiple levels of governments in many countries have mainly ignored or responded superficially, with little to no long-term impact. For decades, federal, provincial, and territorial governments have successively promised to increase senior and Indigenous communities' quality of life.

Substantive talks rarely occur between governments and countries to produce clear strategies and action plans to be implemented and followed up on to ensure meaningful and beneficial change for young and old everywhere on the planet. Governments ignored past reports and suggestions in dealing with pandemics by not adhering to the "cautionary principles,"[11] resulting in many victims.

Consequently, 'exponential rivalry,' a situation that has plagued humanity for millennia, has dominated political and religious agendas. Though the most common examples are wars, the disappearance of and subjugation of civilizations, and the raping of the planet's resources by ruthless corporations, to name a few, when it comes to Canada's out-dated health care system, exponential rivalry manifests itself in several ways:

- Grotesque greed and wilful disregard of health protocols
- Blind political partisanship
- Political ineptness through inappropriate role models and comments
- Repeatedly making the same mistakes (e.g., opening up prematurely)
- Ignoring best practices of other jurisdictions
- Total disregard for specific sectors of the population

- Wasting resources on developing solutions when existing beneficial results or processes exist in other jurisdictions and are available
- Ignoring scientific facts or acknowledging only the convenient ones

The development of several vaccines to counter the virus's effects is of little comfort to the families and loved ones of the thousands who paid the price with their lives. Without a doubt, these deadly results shattered the Canadian myth that seniors are valued, coupled with the rampant ageism behaviours heard, read, and observed before and during the pandemic by prominent leaders and sadly beyond.

How a country, its governments, and its citizen's treat the elderly does not bode well about people's behaviour as members of the human race.

Among the many highlighted misgivings learned during the COVID-19 pandemic is the presence of an unprecedented number of broken, dysfunctional, detrimental, and out-dated procedures and processes that require an entirely new rethink, re-engineering, or discard. The Canadian health care approach is certainly one at the top of the priorities. Crossing over to the twenty-first century requires rightsizing and modernization.

CHAPTER 5

The Way Forward

Home care support takes on many faces. It is advantageous when a senior is recovering from an illness or surgery and requires help dealing with everyday tasks necessary to their continued recovery from a short-term perspective. From a long-term perspective, home care supports seniors in managing the more challenging and recurring tasks such as the following:

- Food preparation and diet
- Transport to and from appointments and grocery shopping
- Oversee proper medication dosage
- Light housework, including seasonal exterior chores
- Not forgetting companionship, which addresses the long-standing loneliness, further exacerbated during the pandemic

Numerous other services are also available, depending on the expressed needs of seniors. Some will be with volunteers' support, while others will require either family involvement or paid contractors. For instance, outside tasks include mowing the lawn and landscaping or clearing entrances and pathways following a snowstorm. In addition, adult children and extended younger family members living in relative proximity can significantly support their elderly parents, grandparents, and other senior extended family members and neighbours to complete challenging activities.

As mentioned earlier, the documentary *Fast Forward* simulation was designed for immediate and extended family members to demonstrate and experience the challenges linked to ageing, primarily to better understand the challenges their parents/grandparents regularly face and to consider preparing for their future aged self, hopefully. Paraphrasing what one of the speakers shared, "How we age, mirrors how we lived as our younger self."

Seniors and family members should actively explore what types of services are currently available in their neighbourhood. For example, meals-on-wheels, light housekeeping, and volunteer drivers to appointments are extremely useful to help seniors accomplish various tasks and provide a way to connect with other people and reduce loneliness.

Even when seniors still perform these day-to-day tasks, it is prudent and advantageous to plan for future unforeseen circumstances. Registering for these various community support systems is extremely helpful, maybe by having a meal or two delivered via meals-on-wheels or having someone spend one day per month to help with more demanding tasks such as changing sheets, washing windows, etc.

For a senior living alone, these occasional visits provide an opportunity to chat and socialize. Increasing frequencies when needed is far easier than a last-minute request to receive a service or support, especially when faced with a chaotic circumstance.

During a presentation about my journey with my mother, one participant accentuated the high cost of rent and food in the Vancouver area. A moment later, when I suggested they might consider registering to various community support services, such as meals-on-wheels, the person assertively said they did their own cooking and cleaning. Looking around the room, I suggested that by doing so, they might be reducing their food cost with the delivery of a couple of meals weekly.

For ageing parents and their family members, having and being a family caregiver does require serious reflection, conversation, and involvement with pertinent partners. Open and honest discussions and interactions with family members and partners are crucial. For first-timers, the web offers multiple resources.[12]

Honest and respectful conversations highlighting the current and foreseeable challenges and how they can be eliminated or mitigated are critical. Dialogue about the senior's and their family members' expectations, and of course, the benefits for seniors remaining in the home of their choice, will result in buy-in by all parties, a strategy for a comfortable and quality lifestyle, and an agreed-upon action plan.

Provinces and territories supported by the Canadian government would greatly benefit from exploring the health care approach of other countries. Notably, in late 1980, Denmark initiated a massive policy shift by implementing a multidisciplinary home-based care model involving teams of mix-specialists, designed to help older adults age in the home of their choice. It included assessments, preventive care, rehabilitation, and restorative care. Visit Denmark's website for further information and scroll down and click on the video which provides an overview of their innovative approach to elder care. – "The Case for Denmark/

Elder Care"[13] Additionally, a white paper published in September 2019, highlights many creative and innovative processes developed over the past thirty years: "A Dignified Elderly Care in Denmark."[14]

A September 2020 report, "Ageing Well," by Queen's University, clearly illustrates the current status of ageing in Canada. It highlights the impact of the COVID-19 pandemic on seniors and what the future holds if provincial and territorial governments, supported by the federal government, do not get serious about the way forward.[15]

PART 3

Next Steps

The past is the past. We cannot change it. What's important is the lesson we retain and apply as we go forward. Primarily, we based our decisions on the circumstances and situations at that particular time. Good or bad, the best we can do going forward is to learn from these decisions. The present is now, with all its challenges and opportunities.

Generally speaking, most seniors have come to terms with their strengths and challenges, and they have realized that some of the easy tasks and activities aren't simple to do anymore. The challenges tend to show up in body aches after doing them, the time it took to complete, or the inability to complete specific tasks. Sometimes it may come from observations made by family members and friends who have noticed minor changes.

Based on available information from trusted sources and your conclusions, it's probably time to sit down, reflect on everything, and determine the next steps. Waiting for a chaotic situation to unfold is too late.

While we can manage most of our environment, it is prudent to think about the future. Waiting for a challenging situation to confront us as we age may not be the best option. Instead, forward thinking and planning about foreseeable and unforeseeable events while we have the highest level of control and involvement is a wise way forward.

> Recently, while chatting with my sister, she shared that she had broken her leg while moving with her husband, both in their late eighties, a sizable, awkward object down the stairs. As a result, she missed the last step and lost her balance. When asked what lesson she had learned, she laughed and said, "We are not as young as we used to be." No, we aren't.

As we age, it is vital that we come to terms with that reality and seriously think through future actions, tasks, and activities. Engaging in the mindset of cautionary principles should dominate our daily lives. In other words, individuals should always focus and ensure the promotion and protection of their health.

CHAPTER 6

Where the Future Takes You

Our home is, for most of us, where we have lived for a number of years. The amenities, the various services, and friends and family are often more or less in the same neighbourhood. It's comfortable, well located, and where you feel secure—this is why we call it home.

Regardless of the time spent in that home, memories come alive every time we walk in each room. Be it while preparing or having your favourite meal of the day, sitting in your favourite chair, reading a book, or enjoying your preferred beverage on your patio or garden, memories abound.

If not the location itself, then the various family pictures, artwork on the walls, particular furniture handed down from your parents, or items purchased throughout your lifetime that conjure up emotions and memories. These seem to materialize in front of you, the good ones and, unfortunately, some of those you wish you could forget.

Either way, they are part of your history, your experiences, and your life. As we mature in life, certain aspects of our daily/weekly routine or activities become somewhat challenging. Over time, they may become even more so. Yet, whether they occurred outside or inside your home, they served a particular purpose.

Though we are wiser and older, it might be time to consider ways to implement several relatively easy adjustments to make your day-to-day life more comfortable, making sure you can age in the home of your choice.

Several possible alternatives are at your disposal in ensuring your continued well-being and comfort. The options you review should take into consideration your current and possibly future capabilities and health. Whether you choose to remain in your existing home for as long as possible, downsize to a smaller place, move in with a welcoming family member or close friend, or move into a retirement community, you will still have to make some types of adjustments and changes.

"Building on important research by the late Gerald Hodge, a professor emeritus at Queen's University, he describes a series of "push" factors—things likely to trigger relocation—and "pull" factors—conditions where the potential to improve on current conditions are sufficiently strong to inspire a move to a new home…"

…Six 'push factors'

1. Declining health, a reduced ability to manage the daily necessities of life or physical disabilities

2. The need to access equity tied up in one's dwelling, either because of reduced income in retirement or in response to rising costs

3. When rents increase at a greater rate than income

4. Changes in lifestyle or personal circumstance

5. Pressure to relocate closer to their children

6. Isolation from friends and family or declining ambience of the neighbourhood

Four 'pull factors'

1. A wish to reduce the responsibility for maintaining a house or moving to a place that allows more time to travel or undertake other activities.

2. A decision to sell the family home can liberate equity that can be reinvested in a smaller (possibly less expensive) dwelling or reinvested for the purpose of providing a better cash flow to support a different lifestyle.

3. Seeing an opportunity to relocate to a place more conducive to a desired lifestyle.

4. Becoming drawn to an area—possibly within the neighbourhood where they have lived for many years—that possesses a range of housing opportunities and other amenities."[16]

Reflection on these 'push and pull factors' will undoubtedly trigger some responses and ideas and quite possibly identify factors that pertain to your circumstances and environment.

To help you arrive at one or two viable options, I have included a self-assessment tool. Consider completing it. Below are instructions and a short example. You will find a comprehensive blank form in the appendix section.

Instructions for completing the self-assessment tool:

1. Start by making a list of all the things you appreciate and like about your current environment and home.

2. Include every aspect of your well-being, including geographical location, physical, emotional, social, and yes, psychological.

3. Prepare a similar list of all the things you dislike, including the challenges, the limitations, and the inconveniences.

Once the lists are completed, go over each item on the 'like' side and give it a rating of one (being a low 'like') to five (being a high 'like').

> **Note:** Consider using a **green highlighter** pen for items with <u>a four or five</u> <u>ranking</u>, as they are quite important to you.

Repeat the same process on the 'dislike' side, this time using a negative rating—that is, minus one (being a low 'dislike') to a minus five (being a high 'dislike').

> **Note:** Consider using a **red highlighter** pen for items with <u>a minus four or a minus five ranking</u>, as they are situations you prefer eliminating or at least minimizing from your environment.

This analysis, conducted with your spouse, significant other, a family member, or close friend requires total and realistic honesty with yourselves concerning the present and the probable future. Once completed, total each side.

> **Note:** You can repeat this self-assessment yearly or every other year to maintain pertinence.

Which side has the highest total? If it were the 'Likes' side, then it would seem that staying in your current home might be the answer, at the very least, based on your current circumstances. However, implementing some of the adjustments or changes suggested in the following chapters might not only increase your 'Likes' total but also eliminate or mitigate some of the 'Dislikes.'

Should the 'Dislikes' total be the highest, set it aside and read the proposed ideas, adjustments and changes described in the part 4 – Exterior Environment and part 5 – Interior Environment, keeping in mind your appraisal. When ideas or tips pop up to address or resolve a 'Dislike,' then note it on the assessment and continue reading for more, especially when it deals with high minus items you have highlighted. You might discover that several of the ideas and suggestions would minimize or even eliminate many of the concerning 'Dislikes.'

> **Note:** Should the two totals be close to each other, consider including the plus and minus three ranking(s) in your review.

This exercise should help you further narrow down your decision-making process by highlighting all the positive and negative aspects (i.e. the 'Push and Pull factors' described earlier) of your current home and help you decide what best meets your needs and expectations.

Example for Likes and Dislikes Self-Assessment

Current Environment/Home/House: Likes and Dislikes[17]

Likes Appreciated / Convenient	Rate	Dislikes Challenging / Inconvenient	Rate
Close to grocery store	5	Children/grandchildren far	-5
Close to a few friends	3	Few opportunities for social	-4
Home is roomy–three floors	4	Need car for other services	-3
Parking garage	5	No outside space to sit	-5
Mortgage paid	5	City services poor	-4
Can entertain friends	2	Maintenance	-2
House is where I was born	3	Busy area	-2
Hardwood floors	4	Bright nightlights	-2
Park nearby for walks	5	Nosy neighbours	-1
Same phone # for years	1	Safety issues	-1
Etc.		Etc.	
Total	37 28	Total	-29 -18

CHAPTER 7

Remaining in Your Current Home

Okay, so you have decided to stay in your current home. Now what? There are still some challenges and obstacles that need to be addressed or remedied. Should someone in the household be experiencing specific and demanding circumstances which require more focused support, retaining an occupational therapist's services to suggest ways to address such challenges or difficulties is strongly encouraged.

The information you will find in the following chapters comes from my experience as the principal caregiver to my mother, input from other seniors, and reputable research done by various entities. My successes by no means guarantee that you will experience the same outcomes. Your circumstances, financial and physical situation, and environment should dictate what best works for you.

The information provided highlights ideas, suggestions, and tips about the exterior and the interior of your home that you might implement to adapt and transform your environment into a more senior-friendly home. They are potential avenues or triggers for conversation and discussion. In addition, they will often precipitate better ideas and solutions for your specific needs and environment.

Part 4 of this book deals with the exterior environment of your dwelling. Should the exterior of your home fall out of your area of responsibility and you deem that some of the ideas would benefit your safety and quality of life, you certainly could bring these suggestions to the maintenance staff, groundskeeper, or other involved players.

Seniors experience many challenges. Maintaining a thriving, functioning home is undoubtedly one of them. Sadly, though many of us do everything to keep active and healthy, maintaining our strength, abilities, and energy is often quite challenging. When your home's layout limits making changes or adjustments, consider some of the ideas and suggestions of things you can do to the exterior and interior of your environment to make life easier and more manageable for you. They will provide you with various options to consider at no cost, while others require multiple levels of investments.

However, the location of the bedroom, bathroom, and laundry room, will still bring about many challenges that might be difficult to overcome. You can overcome stairs with either a tubular elevator or a stair lift system. However, space limitations might limit such options and require a significant investment that may not be readily available.

Regardless of the size of a house, it still requires cleaning and upkeep. The bigger the house, the more effort and time are needed. Keeping a large house operational so that children can visit for special family events may not be the best option. Everyone leads busy lives, and visits tend to be for the day. They also would prefer not to impose on your daily/weekly routine.

Some years ago, a work colleague of mine bought a much larger house, even though both children had moved away across the country, expecting they, with their growing families, would come and visit regularly. Sadly, their active lifestyle took precedence, and they barely came once a year. She eventually sold the house and moved to their current location.

CHAPTER 8

Involving Family

Once you have done your reflection, I strongly suggest that you involve your closest family members. I can certainly appreciate the challenge of what I am proposing. Independence, control over our lives, and the ability to do what we wish to do when we want to do it are essential to our well-being. Still, consider the other side of the coin. Yes, you want to remain in the home of your choice as long as you can. Great! Is it a viable option?

Why not enlist your children's support and involvement to make that happen? It's a win-win proposition—your peace of mind and theirs. Additionally, hearing directly from you about the challenges you are currently experiencing will help them better understand your perspective and look for ways to support you in having your decision come to fruition.

Unfortunately, this aspect is one of the mishaps of my experience with my mother. The involvement and sharing of information with other family members were at times sketchy. They knew she would live with me; however, the details of her decisions were not all shared, especially some of the challenges and hardships she had been enduring over the last few years. I discovered some through conversations with her live-in caregiver, Denise. However, most of them were unknown until after mother moved in with me, after several months when she felt secure and comfortable enough to share the missing details.

Finding the fortitude and the courage to share what you are experiencing is an essential step for all seniors, regardless of the challenges experienced. Even on delicate or sensitive topics such as personal hygiene issues, medical limitations, estate planning, and end-of-life wishes and expectations, being upfront with family members may be uncomfortable and challenging, both for seniors and family members; however, it should be part of ongoing conversations.

I continued my weekend visits, discussing next steps with Mom and Denise, her live-in companion. During one conversation, when Mom was not present, Denise apologetically shared information that was unknown to me, as Mom had asked her to say nothing about it. She now felt she needed to inform me as the move was eminent. Based on Denise's observations, Mother had been struggling for nearly two years. The freezing winters made it difficult for her to be sufficiently warm and comfortable. Her mobility had significantly reduced due to her eyesight. Mom often sat in silence. When Denise inquired if everything was okay, my mother replied that living in this old house was getting more and more challenging for her. When Denise reminded her of my frequent invitation to move in with me, she mostly said she did not want to be an imposition to anyone.

Whatever your wishes, expectations, or desires, I am sure you want to ensure they are respected, so put those subjects on the table for discussion. I encourage you to be truly honest with yourself and your family. Attractive options and perspectives can come out of your interactions and conversations.

Mother's decision to live in her own home for ten years had prepared both her and me. At the time for her, the move was a significant life change. However, more was to come. The reality that my mother chose to take a decade to reflect and process such a move was undoubtedly a wise decision on her part. Then, the nearly six months to prepare the actual move with everything it involved provided both of us with ample time to internalize emotionally and psychologically this significant life change that would unfold. It was instrumental in ensuring my mother's quality of life, safety, and comfort.

The move went quite well. My sister drove to the farmhouse and brought Mother back to her home for a few days, while family members and close friends lent a hand in loading, unloading, and setting up everything in the new house. I remained home for a few days to ensure she would find her way around her new home. Happily, she figured her way around the various rooms within three days. What helped was having her furniture and accessories set up in the new place. The early evening she arrived in her new home, as I helped with her coat, she, for a moment, thought of being back at the farm. Then her favourite chair and a blazing fire in the fireplace came into focus. At that moment, she knew this would be her new home.

PART 4
Exterior Environment

Many of us have been living in our current home for many years. Though styles, sizes, and locations differ, you probably have been doing all the tasks to maintain your house and surroundings, automatically, without much thought, going about doing what you needed to do in ways that worked for you. Regrettably, these same routines may have gotten somewhat overwhelming and sometimes challenging to complete as time passed. Unfortunately, for various reasons, we often fail to consider making changes or adjustments to our home environment until a mishap occurs or we are unable to complete basic tasks.

The following information highlights ways to ensure that the exterior of your home is devoid of obstacles or situations that might cause a fall.

"Falls are the leading cause of injury among seniors in Canada, experiencing between 20 to 30 percent of falls yearly, leading to 85 percent of injury-related, and 95 percent of hip-fracture hospitalizations, of which 50 percent happened at home."[18]

Depending on your location, circumstances, and yearly seasonal variances, some of these activities may have become difficult to complete. The smaller trees and bushes have grown. Deciduous trees are now higher than the house, and though beautiful most of the time, unfortunately, during the autumn season, they shed their colourful leaves on the roof, in the eavestrough, on the lawn, and garden. What may have taken a couple of hours or less to mow the lawn and care for your flowers, and possibly your vegetable patch, may have become a week or more to complete.

If you live in a colder climate, shovelling the driveway and walkways may have become a significant project. If you feel you can tackle such a task safely, then proceed. However, there may come a time when it might be simply too much. Acceptance of this reality is key. Options to deal with inclement weather will be further highlighted in following chapters.

Almost twenty years ago, I moved into my current home—a single-storey cottage nestled in a quiet rural area. The three-car-length driveway and the house sit on about two acres with another fourteen acres of forest behind. Over the first few years, I cut back some of the trees for firewood, cleared stumps and rocks, and brought in some topsoil to expand the lawn's size. Additionally, I created a dozen flowerbeds, a couple of vegetable patches, and a tiny Zen garden with a nice bench under the trees to meditate and relax. Except for the past two or three years, I enjoyed doing the work required to care for and maintain my property. However, during the past couple of years, I found it much more challenging to complete the work needed to keep the entire area the way I wanted. In addition, preparation and maintenance activities became much more difficult as I got older—for example, raking the copious amount of leaves and broken branches, setting out and storing lawn ornaments, and the spring cleaning, seeding, and planting preparation, not forgetting the snow removal season, especially the thick and heavy section left by the snowplough.

Over the years, I thoroughly enjoyed my property. Mowing the lawn was a great way to relax and forget about the stressors of daily life. But, of course, during the same time, I aged. Many of the activities and responsibilities began to be somewhat overwhelming and demanding. After some minor incidents, I got someone to help out.

I enlisted a friend to help out on weekends with the more challenging tasks. Unfortunately, my pride took the better of me, and I continued doing much of the work. Two years ago, I went overboard. My primary source of heat during the winter is a high-efficiency wood stove. Every August, I call to give my order, delivered in September/October. Depending on the previous winter usage, the neighbouring farmer brings eight to ten face cords in two trips, unloading them in my driveway near the garage. Over several days, I cord about four of them inside the garage and the rest outside along the garage wall. While installing a tarp on the outside stack, I slipped and fell off. Luckily, except for several bruises, I did not break anything. Right there and then, I decided it was time to accept that my abilities were no longer what they were when I moved here. Even though I do everything I can to maintain a healthy lifestyle, I'm now in my seventies, and there are certain limitations I can no longer deny. The incident made me realize that I needed to stop resisting, so I did what I did for my mother during my years as her caregiver; and made some adjustments and meaningful changes to make my life easier.

At the end of Chapter 10, you will find a short example of an exterior checklist that should help you pinpoint potential situations or conditions that might lead to a fall or injury to you and your loved ones. Eliminating or, at best, minimizing risks of injuries is vital. Please do not wait for an accident to happen to address these hazards.

Appendix II is a comprehensive exterior checklist, which can be replicated or copied. I encourage you not to procrastinate on situations that can cause harm to someone. Waste no time in evaluating your exterior environment. Be proactive.

CHAPTER 9

Eliminating or Minimizing Exterior Risk Factors

Walkways and driveways: Keep walkways (includes driveway, garage floor, seasonal or permanent carport, sidewalks, walkways, or paths to all entrances, garden, patio, etc.) free of bumps, holes, cracks, and structural items such as high thresholds, rickety fences, and shaky gates. Remove branches or bushes and any other things that could cause someone to trip and fall. Strategically place solar or motion sensor lights to illuminate frequently used passageways, including steps leading to and from a patio or garden area, not forgetting to make sure handrails are sturdy. Landscaping solar lights will minimize and, in most cases, eliminate risks of injuries, and solid grab bars will ensure stability.

If you have a wood stove or a fireplace, make sure the wood is safely stored in the garage, a lean-to, or a covered outside area, ensuring nothing creates a barrier or an obstacle. For safety reasons, use a set of two metal 2 × 4 rack structures (often available at Rona Hardware[19]) and four pieces of 2" × 4" × 4' treated lumber to stack wood. The plastic log stackers tend to break easily, especially in sub-zero winters, and are not optimal. The market offers small and medium-size log racks for outdoor and indoor use for smaller amounts of wood.

<u>Stairways, handrails, and porches:</u> Ensure stairways to all entrances are in good condition and, where appropriate, fitted with exterior rugged anti-slip strips; solid and unshakable handrails, preferably on both sides; and for added safety, security motion sensor floodlights. When feasible, having a conveniently placed shelf or bench at the main entrance to lay down bags or boxes provides easier access to locked doors. Lever-style door handles facilitate opening doors. A locking system that requires using a key for the locking mechanism will prevent unfortunate situations, such as stepping out to get the mail and the door closing behind you.

However, the inside deadbolt section should be a single-cylinder type that does not require a key to lock. Doorway thresholds should not exceed more than one-half inch, or thirteen centimetres. In cases where it does, see if it can be lowered or changed to a no-step style. Strategically installed solar or battery-powered motion sensor lights, available at your local hardware store, would illuminate the door area and locking mechanism, significantly increasing visibility and access after sundown.

Mail delivery is vital for homebound seniors. The mailbox should be relatively easily accessible. If you have a mail slot in the bottom door, consider getting a small basket installed below the space to catch the mail, preventing the need to pick it up off the floor. Unfortunately, mail slot tend to not be very energy wise.

If you have a mailbox just outside your door, ensure nothing obstructs its access by the mail carrier. Recently developed neighbourhoods often do not have home mail delivery. Instead, homeowners need to go to a centralized location nearby. In such cases, consider getting a letter from your doctor explaining that you are homebound. Prepare a letter requesting the post office permission for direct home delivery and take it to your post office for approval.[20]

Wheelchair accessibility: Rather than changing the entire door structure, consider changing the door's standard hinges to a swing clear or offset model, which can widen clearance by several inches. This low-cost solution will facilitate entry for someone who requires the use of a walking assistance device such as a walker, crutches, mobility scooter, wheelchair (the minimum width required is thirty-six inches), etc. In addition, when a household member requires a walking aid and your home has several steps, an appropriate ramp structure will safely facilitate access to the house. Check for local requirements or bylaws for such a structure. Get several quotes from recognized contractors that provide precise details of the finished product.

Your location: Ensure that your civic number/address stands out and is always visible from the street in case of emergencies. Using a colour that is the opposite of the exterior finish of your house is best as will visually stand out. Some signs can also light up to enhance visibility.

Enlisting support: Maintain or seek help from a family member or a friend for trimming branches, bushes, and trees that might have a destructive impact on power lines and the house's structure during high winds and harsh weather patterns. Then, in late autumn, enlist their support to clean the roof and eavestrough of leaves and debris, taking them away to the roadside for pickup or to an appropriate location. The marketplace does offer a gutter guard that prevents the eavestrough from getting clogged, should this be a financially viable option.

Seasonal preparation: During the warmer season, secure lawn or patio furniture such as chairs, umbrellas, small tables, and other lighter items when not in use and possibly store them securely during extreme weather patterns and the winter season.

> During the years Mom lived with me, I purchased and installed a seasonal sunshade canopy with a table and a few chairs on the deck. I anchored it with two-inch screws on the wooden floor. Because the deck was quite large, it provided a place for my mother to sit during the summer months, with ample space around it to put several planters of flowers. Unfortunately, every year, one can observe various types of unsecured structures blown away by strong winds. Anticipating such climate events will prevent loss and possibly injury to individuals.

Challenging tasks: Tasks such as window washing, minor repairs, lawn and garden preparation and maintenance, snow removal, and bringing the weekly trash and recycling to the roadside can be daunting. Asking for the support of family members or neighbourhood friends will alleviate the most demanding activities. Contractors can certainly reduce and possibly eliminate this burden, thus minimizing the possibilities of injuries or mishaps. Consult with friends or neighbours to obtain the contact information of reliable contractors.

CHAPTER 10

Minimizing Expenses and Enlisting Support

Bartering or exchanging services can be an option for seniors looking for ways to limit their expenses. You may have been a teacher, a landscaper, a plumber, a lawyer, a well-versed home repairperson, an accountant, an HR professional, a consultant during your career, etc. These are skills that friends, neighbours, and small businesses often need. Your experience and *savoir faire* provide them with direction, guidance, and support. List all the skills, talents, and abilities you possess that you are comfortable practising and happy to share with others as a means of payment with friends, neighbours, family members, and even small contractors who take over the more challenging tasks around the house.

Another possibility is to chat with your neighbours concerning their challenges and needs. For example, you might have the skills or abilities they need and vice versa.

> In my sister's area, interested neighbours and friends created and shared a list of names and contact information that included the types of skills, tasks, or activities they were open to doing for members on the list in exchange for services they needed or for a token remuneration.

For minor repairs dealing with plumbing or electrical issues, when landscaping maintenance and snow removal are required, pooling your needs can be helpful during negotiations to obtain better pricing. Often, trade professionals tend to charge a base fee for the call plus an amount per hour for the service.

The services provided in the exact general location reduce their travel costs. In such instances, you might be able to get a small discount on the hourly fee and for sure have the base fee split among those involved, with the hourly price paid by each party involved.

My sister and her husband banded together with several other seniors on their street. As a result, they negotiated a much better price for landscaping activities and snow removal with a contractor during the winter months. Exterior window washing was also something they dealt with. At first, there were only five or six participants. Now there are several dozen neighbours involved, and their cost is fifty dollars for all exterior windows, equipment, and cleaning materials included.

My experience caring for my mother and my life changes form the basis for these ideas and suggestions. The intent is to encourage you to make a concerted effort to analyze all aspects and determine if any issues could cause harm to you and your loved ones. Additionally, you might be experiencing other challenges linked to the outside of your home—for instance, more energy-wise windows or the replacement of roof shingles.

These significant improvements, of course, require substantial investment and should be considered in the decision-making of remaining in your current home or downsizing, as further discussed in a later chapter.

Instructions for Exterior Checklist

- Check each descriptor for the various exterior areas. I have added blank spaces on the entire checklist in Appendix II for areas or circumstances specific to your environment.

- For each descriptor, determine if the area is risk-free. If yes, write OK or put a ✓ in the 'Risk Free' column, then move to the next item on the list.

- If not risk-free, then indicate actions required in one of the three categories as follows:

  - <u>I can take action</u> - What will I do to fix it?
  - <u>Need support from family and friends</u> - Who can help me fix it?
  - <u>Investigate probable contractor</u> - Research or get a reference for a reputable and reliable contractor/supplier.

Sample Exterior Checklist—
Eliminating/Minimizing Risks

Risk Free	Description of area	I can take action	Need support from family and friends	Investigate probable contractor
OK	Walkways and driveways			
✓	Bushes and branches			
	Proper lighting at entrances	Buy		
	Solid stairways, handrails, and porch		Son to help	
	Anti-slip strips— exterior style	Buy		
	Motion sensor lights/solar lights		Neighbour to help	
	Bench/table at main entrance			Order a bench online
	Etc.			
	Etc.			
	Etc.			
	Etc.			

PART 5
Interior Environment

Once the exterior space is free of clutter and hazards, ensuring safe access and mobility, it is now time to turn your attention to the areas inside your house to provide a more senior-friendly environment. As mentioned in a previous chapter, 50 percent of falls experienced by seniors occur in the home. It is, therefore, crucial that seniors make every attempt to ensure that all potential precarious situations be eliminated or at best minimized, as they too often cause falls.

I will work my way through the various typical areas or rooms in the house, highlighting ideas that should minimize and sometimes eliminate hazardous situations. Some of the suggestions do not require spending money, just some easy adjustments or reorganization. Others might require minimal expenses, and some may need a more significant investment on your part.

However, it is up to you to decide if the return on investment is worthwhile for you at this point.

In chapter 18, I will address the option of downsizing from a larger home to something smaller or more convenient to your needs, especially when the cost of beneficial senior-friendly changes of the current home outweighs the feasibility of such adjustments.

Depending on your level of comfort and mobility, you should be able to make some of these adjustments or changes yourself. However, in some cases, it would be prudent to enlist the help of a family member, a friend, and even a reputable contractor.

At the end of this part, Chapter 16, you will find a tool in Appendix III—'Interior Checklist—Eliminating/Minimizing Risks.' It essentially covers all the room-by-room ideas, suggestions, and tips highlighted in the following six chapters. It should support you in identifying hazardous situations that could be harmful to you and your loved ones.

CHAPTER 11

Entrances

Though different words describe that particular area (entryway, foyer, vestibule), it requires extra attention for several reasons:

- A well-lit entrance with easily accessible switches or equipped with motion sensor lights will enhance safety. The floors must be free from any obstructions or situations that may cause a fall. Unless fitted with double-sided sticky tape or a rubberized backing to prevent slippage, you should remove area rugs. Some cultures use ornate rugs as a wall decoration. Should you have a superior quality area rug, hanging it would allow you to continue appreciating it safely. Slippery flooring materials, especially when wet, can cause falls. To ensure safety, utilize anti-slip strips or add a non-skid additive to floor finish.

- Having a second door (often called a storm door) that locks, with possibly a top window/screen through which you can quickly see when someone is at the door, will increase safety and security. When this is not possible, doors should have a slide chain lock or swing bar (similar to hotels), an eye-level small half-moon window, or peephole (less expensive and easy to install—you can find helpful videos on YouTube) so you can safely ascertain who is at the door.

- Some older houses may not have a doorbell. Local hardware stores carry affordable wireless doorbell systems with adjustable volume to address that need without having expensive wiring completed by a licenced professional. If so inclined, the marketplace has camera technology that permits you to see who is at your door without having to open the door. Maintaining locked doors is of the utmost importance, regardless of where you reside, urban or rural. Opening the door to strangers is not desirable unless you have requested their presence or ordered something online. Ask to see proper identification, regardless of who is at the door and what clothing or uniform they are wearing.

- As mentioned in the previous chapter, a lever-style door handle facilitates manoeuvring doors; however, be aware that loose clothing or handles of bags or purses can get hooked during movement. Minimize unsafe situations when entering or exiting the house or moving about in and around the house. Take your time! If the phone is ringing, the answering system will take care of it, or they can call back.

- As suggested for the main exterior entrance, placing a small bench or chair at the entrance area to lay down parcels or other items as you get ready to go out or upon your return will free up your hands and ensure trouble-free accessibility and movement in that area. It also makes putting on and removing footwear comfortable and safe. Note that proper footwear is essential in securing safe mobility both around the house as well as outside. Flip-flops, sandals, and other similar soft-style footwear, though comfortable and convenient, do not maintain stability and do not appropriately support your ankles/feet, which, unfortunately, can lead to injuries.

> During the years I cared for my elderly mother, I found in a local store low-heel shoes, slippers, and even winterized overshoes that securely closed with a Velcro strap.

- Many entrances tend to have a closet or area to hang coats and store footwear and other frequently used items such as umbrellas. While on the subject of umbrellas, a stand holder with a drip tray will prevent slippage on a wet floor. Ensure effortless access to the closet by not overfilling it with items not used during certain seasons. Storing seasonal clothing and footwear in different closet spaces is often the safest option. For situations where there is no light fixture in the closet, consider obtaining one (or more) battery-powered motion sensor lights at your local hardware store to increase visibility and access.

- When residing in a colder climate, having a small container of sand or non-corrosive salt on the floor of the closet to spread on slippery steps will help you and visitors prevent falls and injury.

- Sometimes, as we age, some of our senses diminish, such as hearing or sight. For example, consider devices equipped with flashing lights or vibrations to inform occupants of persons attempting to announce their presence.

> My current home has two front entrances. I put easy-to-see and easy-to-read signage on one of the entrances that directs visitors, deliveries, and so on to the side door, which is equipped with a wireless doorbell that indicates the presence of someone I can see before opening the door.

- While on the subject of hearing, have you checked out your local provider of hearing aids? Today's technology has come a long way. After resisting the idea for several years, I got my first pair shortly after New Year's 2020, and I have no regrets. Such an improvement! I can now hear all the beautiful bird melodies and group conversations.

CHAPTER 12

Kitchen/Dining Area

The kitchen is an area with several risk factors. Constant vigilance and awareness are continuous requirements. Electric, natural, or propane gas stoves can accidentally cause intense flames. Coupled with water, sharp objects and breakable kitchenware interact; there is an opportunity for injury.

The kitchen is where people spend a significant portion of their time. Whether it is to prepare meals, put away groceries, or enjoy each other's company and conversation over a meal. In some cases, especially for special occasions and family gatherings, the dining room becomes the main space to eat and enjoy joyful conversations.

Here are a few adjustments you can easily make, on your own or with the support of a family member, which would increase your day-to-day comfort, with the ability to adjust to occasional changing demands:

- First and foremost, proper lighting is essential in the kitchen. When replacing bulbs, consider the energy efficient LED "Daylight" types, which provide a brighter glow and usually last longer. Keep your receipts, as a small percentage may fail.

- A comfortable area with a reliable and even surface is a great feature to have in the kitchen during food preparation. It could be a table or a kitchen island with space for a comfortable chair or stool. For tiny kitchen space, the marketplace offers wall-mounted foldaway tables for smaller areas, which, when not in use, take up little space and often have a secondary benefit.

- Harsh cleaning products should be removed and replaced with less toxic and more environmentally friendly products. Many are corrosive and could harm users.

- Always ensure anti-skid flooring.

Over several weeks, maybe a month or two, note all the kitchenware, utensils, food items, and small appliances or equipment you frequently use and their specific location in the kitchen or nearby. Check out the samples of the review forms for the kitchen at the end of this chapter. Comprehensive blank forms are available in Appendixes III and IV.

Once you have done this analysis, mobility permitting or with the support of a family member or friend, move the daily/weekly items to the most conveniently accessible shelves in all your cupboards and pantry, eliminating the need for risky stepladders.

Should you still require a stepladder, please consider using a sturdy type where the third step is approximately twenty-four inches (sixty centimetres) above the ground, that folds flat for storage yet, when open, and has a solid handle to hold on to that stands about forty-two inches (about a hundred centimetres) above the ground floor. A word of caution: You should make every attempt to eliminate the need for a stepladder, as it is potentially risky, regardless of your mobility.

Next, store all the less used or special occasion items on the least convenient and more problematic to reach shelves. Then, when needed during special events, a family member or friend can move them to accessible counters or tables.

Don't forget that drawers and cupboard are more comfortable to open using medium to large D-shaped handles. This style eliminates the possibility of getting caught on the drawer knobs. If doing some kitchen renovations, consider handless drawers and cupboard doors, or the type that closes and opens automatically with a gentle push. No handles or knobs are required.

Doing this process, you will undoubtedly discover that you have items you haven't used in a long while, maybe years. In such a case, you could either sell them or give them away to family members, friends, or a charity of choice. Please discard past-due food items, as they are a health issue.

Over our lifetime, we accumulate various items and memorabilia that have sentimental value to us. However, in today's fast-paced world, younger family members and generations may not use them. They tend to have a minimalistic lifestyle, thus facilitating mobility to other parts of the country or the world. Instead of keeping them for later distribution, please make a list; share it with family members to determine interest. Give these things out now when they need them.

After the first ten years of caring for my mom in the family home as per her wishes, she accepted my long-term offer to come and live with me. The family home, built around 1888, had fifteen mostly large rooms, of which seven were bedrooms. When moving her things to a smaller house, making choices specifically for our needs became the main challenge —one main floor with everything she needed and a finished basement. During the planning for the move, mainly due to the height of the older farmhouse ceilings, which were an average of ten feet high (a bit over three meters), some pieces of furniture remained in the house for the future occupant, my older brother. Both Mother and I were good cooks, resulting in two fully equipped kitchens. We resolved the duplication of many items by keeping the most practical and newer things from either one of our kitchens. What was no longer needed was offered to family members or given to charitable organizations. Some items were past their time, like the early-twentieth-century toaster, an appliance that I saw as dangerous more than anything else. Even today's young millennials would not be interested in using it. However, I discovered that some of these older antique models might be worth hundreds of dollars for collectors researching the web. Maybe I lost out on a few dollars.

In the downsizing chapter 18, I will share my approach to choosing what you may keep and what you might not. On the topic of small appliances and kitchenware, consider the following options:

- If you are looking to upgrade or replace your pop-up toaster, look into a toaster-style oven with a timer where, when you open the door, the tray comes out to facilitate placing items you wish to toast or bake. The ringing tells you it's ready. This feature will reduce the danger of burning yourself, of course, using a pair of tongs, potholder, or mitt to remove heated items. Today's model can also be used to bake small to medium-size items.

- Boiling water with the use of a kettle is much safer than using a pot. If you intend on replacing an older one, explore the type that sits on a base. Once it shuts off after boiling the water, you can easily remove it and pour the water to make some tea without having a dangling electrical wire that could get caught somewhere and cause an injury.

- Coffee-making technology has come a long way over the last several decades. If you are a coffee enthusiast, you might look into one of the many models that uses recycling capsules or a model that utilizes a thermos type of pot, which keeps the coffee hot without burning the coffee, which can be off-putting. Smaller models will brew one cup on demand. Others use either the capsule or your preferred ground mixture, sometimes called "two in one."

- If you are a tea drinker, there is also a very convenient teapot style with a removable tubular filter. You put your tea leaves in the filter and pour the hot water into the pot. Once the tea has steeped to your preference, you can remove the filter, letting it drain off the hot water before emptying the leaves in a small compost container. Leaf tea is better for you—unfortunately, the plastic packets of tea leach micro-plastic, which are detrimental to your health.

- Depending on your cooking style and needs, a microwave can be a helpful appliance in the kitchen. It must be placed on a counter or attached to the underside of the cupboard. When positioned higher, there is always the danger of spillage that could cause burns while removing food from the microwave. At the counter level, it facilitates the operation and minimizes the risk of injury.

When Mom moved in with me, I used a button-style microwave for some things, usually heating food or a beverage. To make it easier for her to warm the pre-prepared lunches I made for her, I figured out that two minutes was perfect to have the right temperature without burning her lips. I then installed a piece of thick cardboard to cover all the buttons except the two, the zero, and the start.

One day, while attempting to heat a muffin, she mistakenly pressed the zero button three times, which resulted in twenty minutes of reheating, way too much for the intended goal, which resulted in a carbonized snack. After that, I found a microwave with dials instead of buttons, which I quickly adapted to prevent turning the dial further than two minutes, and when I was there, I could remove the stopper and use the required time needed.

Today's technology is further advanced. You only have to press a number like one or two to set the cooking time to one or two minutes. The evolution of various recipes has also increased the usage of microwaves. For instance, I can make myself a small bread bun in less than two minutes using a keto approach. Nonetheless, the dial-style microwave is still available on the market.

- Ensure that you safely store, donate, or dispose of duplicate or unused small appliances and other kitchen items such as utensils (including knives), pots, pans, mixing bowls, etc. Doing so will make your cupboards more spacious and much easier to access what you seek.

- Space permitting, a "Lazy Susan" in a cabinet can be helpful to store and access cookware.

- When your children have moved on to their own homes, consider using smaller, lightweight cookware to prepare your meals. A "Reacher Grabber" can be a helpful tool in the kitchen and other areas of your home. If you purchase this, I suggest getting the higher quality, undoubtedly being more robust and convenient.

- For larger appliances, if you want to change or upgrade to an Energy Star refrigerator, look into the model where the freezer section is on the bottom. The most often used refrigerated section is at the top, whether with a single door or the side-by-side French doors, making accessibility much more convenient. As for a stove, especially when someone is experiencing reductions in their vision, some models are easier to clean and feature a red light that lights up on the stovetop front to warn you that it's hot. Having the stove and cooktop controls on the front of the unit is much safer. That location eliminates the need to reach over hot elements or heated food items.

- For added security, an ABC-rated fire extinguisher should be readily accessible in case of emergency, placed approximately five to six feet (one and a half to two metres) from the stove. For safety reasons, please conduct an annual pressure gauge check to ensure it is within operational guidelines. For homes with other sources of fire, like a stove or fireplace, a fire extinguisher should also be in proximity, essential when on another floor.

- As previously mentioned, anti-slip strips or small thin rugs with a rubberized back might be helpful to reduce the danger of slipping, especially around the sink and main food preparation areas.

- The size of containers that we handle frequently can cause unfortunate incidents. I respect that one can save money when buying items in large quantities, such as large jars of condiments, jumbo size boxes of cereal, large containers of milk and juice, or other food items. However, handling them can be tricky. As we get older, we may lose some of our tactile abilities as well as strength. It could be arthritis or other similar ailments.

- Based on your eating habits, buying smaller containers of perishable food items is wiser and safer for your health. In contrast, other things with a longer shelf life can be purchased in larger quantities, as long as you can handle and store them safely.

> When Mom moved in with me, I had to rethink my purchasing approach. Mother had arthritis, so she had difficultly picking up items such as a typical jar of jam, mayonnaise, or a litre (34 ounces) of milk. In certain parts of Canada, milk comes in several types of packaging. One of them is a four-litre bag containing three individually packed 1.33-litre (45 ounces) milk bags. When needed, you put the smaller bag into a specialized oval jug, cut a little corner of the bag, and pour. This approach keeps unopened packs fresher longer. Unfortunately, Mother could not pick these bags up, so I started buying smaller 500 ml cartons that she could easily handle. For condiments, jams, and other items, I purchased the smaller jars, and when I used them, I never closed the cover too tightly. Otherwise, she could not open the lid.

- Regardless of the location of sinks in the house, lever or touch-less style faucets are much easier to manoeuvre than turn-style faucets. To prevent scalding yourself, consider reducing the temperature of your water heater to between 120° and 125° Fahrenheit or between 48° and 52° Celsius. A slightly lower temperature might also be advisable.

Kitchen counters and adjoining spaces should be kept clear of unused cookware and all refrigerated food items stored once finished with them. This also applies to certain food containers that once opened, with content still to be used, should be refrigerated. Such a habit will minimize spoilage and risk of incidents. If you have house pets, then food and water bowls should be placed in out-of-the-way areas. Some pets tend to push bowls around. Consider getting a size-appropriate and heavier elevated stand that holds both food and water bowls, yet is harder for your pet to push toward high passageways.

Dining areas vary from one home to another. For example, some dwellings use the kitchen table for most meals and a formal dining room for more prominent gatherings of family and friends. In smaller homes, it could be one or the other. That is to say that your kitchen space can accommodate a large table for small and large groups and as such, there is no dining room. In other cases, the kitchen space may not have space for a table.

It is always safer for everyone that movement toward and around the table is accessible and obstruction-free. In addition, wood, tile, or similar hard surfaces in the kitchen and dining area make it easier to sit or stand up, especially if the legs of the chairs have small felt pads, which requires less effort to manoeuvre, as well much easier to clean and maintain.

The kitchen table could accommodate our entire family with a few places to spare, where I grew up. The more formal dining room had an antique oak table with lion's paws that opened up to seat twelve to fourteen people. It was used during holidays when extended family members were present. When my mother moved in with me, the kitchen could only accommodate a small table opposite the cooking area. However, it was easily accessible upon walking into the kitchen. When my siblings and their families came over for various gatherings, we used the dining room. Because it was also near the patio door that led to a large deck, when not in use, I positioned the dining room table closer to the wall, facilitating movement to and from the deck obstruction-free.

Please pay special attention to decorative objects, such as planters, floor lamps, picture frames, shelves with decorative knick-knacks, etc. They may stick out, including outwardly chair and table legs, causing someone to either trip and fall or hurt themselves when bumping into these objects.

The following section will provide you with the information to conduct a review of everything you currently have in your kitchen. This tool will help you identify frequently used items and rarely (sometimes never) used items. In addition, such a process will create more space and allow you to store things on easily accessible shelves.

Instructions to complete the review of the kitchen (please read the instructions before starting your review):

- Using the "most used" checklist, for a month or more, list the names of the kitchenware, utensils, and small appliances you frequently use—that is, daily, weekly, or monthly.

- Writing down their location—that is, cupboards, pantry, or elsewhere—with a pencil will make things easier for you when you take action.

- As you complete this first checklist, write on the "rarely/never" list the kitchenware, utensils, and small appliances you do not seem to use, noting down in pencil their location.

- Next, at an opportune time, place all the "rarely/never" used items on a table and determine what you will do with them as per the following criteria:
  - Keep for a special occasion
  - Give away to family and friends[21]
  - Sell online or at a garage sale
  - Recycle or trash

- Once you have created space, place the frequently used items on easily accessible shelves in your cupboards or pantry and the special occasion items in the newly created space.

- The rationale for using a pencil for location is to make the future easier. As you put away your daily, weekly, and monthly used items, erase to the old place and write the new location as a memory jogger for the future. Remember, most of these items have been in a specific area for years. This document will help you find your things faster until it becomes second nature.

Sample Review – Kitchenware, Utensils, Small Appliances

Most Used Kitchenware, Utensils, Small Appliances, Etc.		
Items	**Location**	**Frequency** D = Daily W = Weekly M = Monthly
Mixing bowls	Under counter shelf	W
Mixing spoons, spatulas, etc.	Right drawer	D
Waffle maker	Pantry	M
Toaster	Corner counter	D
Etc.		

Sample Review –
Kitchenware, Utensils, Small Appliances

Rarely/Never Used Kitchenware, Utensils, Small Appliances, Etc.		
Items	**Location**	**Next steps** SO = Special Occasions Give = G Sell = S Trash = T
Bread maker	Under counter shelf	G or S
Chocolate fountain	Garage shelf	S or T
Large wooden salad bowl	Garage shelf	SO
Broken beyond repair kettle	Pantry	Recycle/Trash
Etc.		

CHAPTER 13

Living and Family room / Den / Office Area

As we get older, another challenge that creeps up on us is mobility. It is therefore vital to maintain an active lifestyle to keep our mobility to its highest capacity. Activity is medicine. Nevertheless, that can sometimes be challenging, especially when we are experiencing specific difficulties.

Unfortunate circumstances might be a trigger to review your environment. It would be advantageous to have a family member or friend help you look at your furniture setup to identify items that are no longer used that might create a mobility hazard. Give them away, sell them, or call a charitable organization that will be pleased to come over and take them off your hands to repurpose for people who appreciate and need such items. When dealing with Habitat for Humanity, for example, not only will they come and pick up the items, when they repurpose or resell them, you may receive a charitable donation receipt.

Placing furniture to allow ample space to move about will minimize tripping situations or needlessly bumping into them, which is especially useful when someone in the household uses an assistive device. Consider keeping a small table next to your favourite sitting area, which is useful for books, magazines, and remotes for your entertainment devices, reading glasses while enjoying conversations with other family members, or watching television. Maybe a small table lamp or a floor lamp can provide you with necessary lighting when reading. Please resist the urge to use three-legged tables, as they can be wobbly and not as stable as people think when used as a support to sit or stand, and they can also tip over.

If you have either a fireplace or woodstove, ensure all flammable furniture or other items are placed at a safe distance when rearranging the area. Having a small metal pail with a cover and handle to take ashes away is critical to your safety. Depending on how much you use it, consider having a chimney sweep contractor do a yearly professional cleaning. Years of soot accumulation will possibly double and sometimes triple the cost of cleaning. A chimney fire would create an undesired and potentially harmful situation to your home and your health. An ABC fire extinguisher relatively near a fireplace or stove will increase safety during emergencies. Please discard ashes in a metal trash can with a solid lid, storing them outside in a safe place.

Today's telecommunications technology has gone through major changes in the last twenty years. Cellphones or mobiles tend to be present in most households, offering convenience, incoming messaging opportunities, and easy access. The well-known telephone landline has also gone through beneficial and useful improvements. For instance, the convenience of linking two or three portable cordless units located in different parts of the home and incoming answering option eliminates the need to hurry to answer when a call comes in, thus minimizing injuries.

Ensure you choose a model with the most prominent number buttons and the capacity to pre-program numbers such as 911, family members, etc. During an emergency, a pad of paper and pen with your address, situated near the phone, would be helpful. In such cases, we can sometimes panic and momentarily forget vital information. In Canada, most phone providers now offer the free option to limit and, in most cases, eliminate unwanted calls from intrusive robocalls. Just ask your provider how it works and have it enabled. It also works for mobile devices.

Take your time walking in and out of carpeted rooms, as there may be a high threshold that could cause you to trip. Wood floors tend to be safer; however, be careful of spilled liquids that might render them slippery. As mentioned earlier, eliminate area rugs and, if possible, thick-pile rugs, which can be detrimental when walking from one area to another. If you desire wall-to-wall carpet due to warmth, then explore the low-pile type to determine if it meets your needs. Having double-sided sticky tape on area rugs could help; however, depending on the thickness, it might be safer to remove those situated in all pathways to access and move about the room.

Anything on the floors that tends to be less visible is unsafe. Decide on the usefulness and requirement of such items and minimize or eliminate the risk when another alternative is possible. For example, phone cords, electrical extensions, and cell phone charging cables should be placed along walls or attached to a particular furniture side. Your local hardware store carries small self-sticking clips that will make this easy.

The web highlights video clips, often found by searching for "life hacks," on safely storing cables and extensions. As previously mentioned, proper footwear is critical to ensure safety and minimize falling or tripping incidents when walking about your home.

Other possible areas of interest are upper floors and basement areas, depending on the type of house. Regardless, solid handrails, preferably on both sides, significantly improve safety when using stairs. With the help of family members and friends, rearrange rooms to concentrate living requirements to the main floor, without having to manoeuvre stairs, unless they have chosen to invest in one of the different styles of lift devices.

The living areas mentioned above require appropriate lighting. Blinds, curtains, and other window coverings should be open during daylight hours. Given the seasonal changes of daylight, individual on-off timers for lamps can be easily programmed and installed to come on at the right time, thus ensuring straightforward accessibility to rooms to prevent incidents.

You can also purchase LED rechargeable nightlights that provide a low light glow in the trickier areas of the house and activate during power outages. Another option to address lighting is to look into larger motion sensor lights that light up when sitting on the side of your bed in the middle of the night, while other lights illuminate the area as you make your way to your next destination.

One night, after my mother moved in with me, I was sleeping downstairs and was awakened by her calling out for me. I got up, and when I attempted to turn the light on the nightstand, I realized there was a power outage. I quickly reached for the flashlight out of a drawer and headed upstairs, finding Mom in the dark, sitting on the side of her bed, wanting to go to the bathroom. I guided her using the flashlight, waited outside the door, and then took her back to her bedroom.

After that situation, I wondered what might have happened had I been away on business. So I set out to find a solution. Motion sensor lights were discovered, bought, and installed within a few days. As she sat up, the light went on, she would walk into the corridor toward the bathroom, and another light turned on, all the way to the bathroom and the kitchen area. I knew then, at least as far as her accessibility was concerned, Mother would be safe.

For added safety, I installed the button on her night table of a wireless doorbell, putting the ring section in my bedroom, should she require my help in the future.

Closet space should have interior lights to facilitate storing and retrieving items. On occasion, because of their location, you might have to purchase battery-powered motion sensor lights that can be either screwed or stuck to the wall and would turn on upon opening the closet door.

The same item is also valuable for illuminating floors or bottoms of staircases situated away from light fixtures.

My living room and bedroom are in a part of the house that is two steps lower than the rest. At the time I purchased the home, this situation was no issue. However, as I got older, I realized and accepted that in the middle of the night, this could cause a fall. I talked about it with my friend and even looked up on the web to see what I could find, yet with no luck.

Eventually, about two or three weeks later, my friend came in from work and gave me a small box. He had purchased a small three-inch-square LED battery-powered motion-activated light. He even installed it for me (stick-on or screwed in). The bright light turns on when I get within three feet (one metre) of the steps.

Smoke detection devices on all floors, including the basement, are a must and required in most jurisdictions. Radon detectors might be helpful; however, before investing in such a device, consider having radon levels tested to determine the need. Whether you have a fireplace or efficiency stove and burn wood or wood pellets or not, you should have a carbon monoxide (CO) detector, as they are required in most Canadian jurisdictions. Some models also include the smoke detection feature. If you have an inside garage, never leave the car running because this will create toxic carbon dioxide gases. It's an excellent habit to annually replace the batteries of all warning devices, clocks, and battery-powered lights.

One option is to pick a specific date, such as your birthday, when daylight savings time ends, or any other significant date. Depending on the device, some require changing twice a year or more. Rechargeable batteries and charging devices can eliminate the continuous need to remember purchasing and safely disposing of regular batteries. If using natural gas for cooking or other gas devices, depending on the age of the appliance, they can produce methane gases. A methane detector test could identify possible issues.

One of these areas may possibly also be used as an office where you have your computer/laptop, a printer, a work desk and chair, a phone, and maybe some books. The features and suggestions mentioned so far also apply to your work area, especially having a comfortable chair and excellent lighting. It is easy to leave things here and there; however, a small filing cabinet or box will save you time searching for specific information. Some people may prefer to use technology, storing their information electronically in the "cloud." [22]

I'm old school. Every piece of information is filed alphabetically for ease of search. Payment dates are entered on my laptop's calendar to ensure timely processing to escape expensive interest charges, even if late by one day or short changed your payment by a few pennies.

A few years back, I reorganized my office space. Going over the many books purchased over fifty years, I decided to consolidate by topic and identify those I knew I would continue to refer to and those I would not. Some were business-related; some were novels; others fell into different genres. The result was four medium-size boxes. I brought those with me to a book fair when I promoted my memoir – *Lasting Touch – a Mother and Son's Journey of Joy, Challenges, Sadness, and Discovery*. They were between 25¢ and $1 each. I sold about half of them, and the money went to my favourite charity—the rest of them went to my local library.

CHAPTER 14

Bedrooms

Moving your bedroom to the main floor close to a full bathroom is the best option if you have space. Regardless, when your home configuration does not make that feasible, ensure that bedrooms have clear and obstruction-free passageways, especially during the night should you have to make your way to the bathroom. Strategically placed nightlights are critical. If the brightness hinders your sleep, have working flashlights in a drawer or on your night table in case of a power outage. All pieces of furniture that are rarely or never used should be moved elsewhere or given away. Enlist the help of a family member for friends for that task.

As mentioned in the living room chapter, store all phone, charging, and extension cables along the wall or behind larger furniture pieces. If you have area rugs, ensure they will not move or slip, using anti-slip strips or made with rubberized undercoating. As you enter a room, easily accessible light switches are critical. You might even consider using rocker-style instead of toggle-style controls. If the design of rooms does not include accessible switches, then install motion sensor lights.

The height of the bed is also an important aspect of safety. When too low, it is a struggle to get out of bed. It is not easy to sit on the side while getting ready to go to bed when too high. Explore the option of adjusting the height to your comfort level. The marketplace offers various bed risers as well as other safety devices for different rooms of the house.[23]

If the electrical outlets are standard, you probably find them to be low or difficult to reach. Instead of retaining an electrician to reposition them for your convenience, consider purchasing quality power bars with a surge protector. You can position the power bar with extra outlets to a more convenient height and accessible location using appropriate fasteners. Be careful about overloading an outlet with too many devices, in other words resist filling every plug-in space.

When your house has a full bathroom and a family room or den on the main floor, then consider getting some help to move your bedroom to that area, thus eliminating the stairs.

Soon after arriving in her house, the stairs to her bedroom were a significant challenge. Luckily, the main floor had a full bathroom, and next to it, my father's old office, and adjoining that room was the TV room. So with the help of my brothers and Denise, we moved the TV and her favourite chair with an extra one, a small table, and a floor lamp into the office space, which was quite spacious. Then we repainted the TV room and got a beautiful light green wall-to-wall low pile carpet, some lovely curtains for the two large windows, and a matching bedspread, all as per Mother's suggestions. Finally, we moved down to the main floor her bed, a wardrobe, a dresser for her clothes, and a couple of chairs, decorating the walls with the pictures that adorned her upstairs bedroom.

If that option is impossible and manoeuvring the stairs is a challenge, consider the following:

- First, how you have tackled stairs all your life may no longer be safe for you, given various situations. Though you are still relatively mobile, the stair issue can be daunting. Staircases must always be well illuminated and obstruction-free. One way you could tackle a set of stairs is to hold on to the banister, preferably on both sides and come down backwards as if you were coming down from a ladder.

- Assistive devices have gone through significant evolution and development over the past decade. Scandinavian countries are well known for developing valuable and beneficial instruments. One of these is the Assisted Stairwalker, which is now available in Canada. Follow the link[24] for an informative video clip on its utilization. This innovative assistive device helps individuals of any age who can still tackle stairs in both directions and wishes to feel safe while remaining active.

- If your circumstances are beyond these approaches, the market offers alternatives such as a tubular vacuum style elevator[25] or a chair lift system.[26] Both have benefits and disadvantages and require a substantial investment.

CHAPTER 15

Full Bathroom / Half Bathroom

Generally speaking, most bathrooms have tiled flooring for ease of cleaning. Newer homes often have heated floors for additional comfort. I have seen some with wall-to-wall low-pile carpets. Here are some ideas and suggestions to increase the level of comfort and security and reduce risks:

- If you have an area rug near the sink and around the toilet, as well as a bathmat, ensure that they either have anti-slip strips or rubberized underside to prevent slipping. Ensure they are not too thick, as the height difference between the floor and the rug can cause one to trip. With wall-to-wall carpeting, remove the heavy-pile rug, installing a lower pile rug instead to prevent tripping and falling. Be careful of the height of the threshold at the entrance. It ought to be as low as possible and, hopefully, level.

- The age of your toilet might be a model that stands lower, thus making it harder to sit or stand up.

Buying a new higher model and hiring a plumber to install it will be costly. Fortunately, the marketplace offers an easily installed raised seat extender with or without arms that lifts the toilet level by about three to four inches (seven to ten centimetres), depending on the manufacturer's design.[27]

- Should this type of raised seat not be required, another safety option is having a solidly installed grab bar near the toilet. Bathroom tissue should be easily accessible to prevent overextension. The toilet's location might be awkwardly distant from accessible tissue paper; therefore, purchasing a freestanding bathroom tissue holder will facilitate access, located as close or far as you desire.

Based on the age of your bathroom fixtures, the sink may not have a space to put items such as a toothbrush, a non-breakable glass, etc. The following are a few ways to address this issue:

- A small wall cabinet positioned above the sink or a small shelf with or without a mirror
- Accessible well-anchored towel racks that can be used as grab bars
- A small table or multi-shelf organizer adjoining the sink
- A wall-mounted soap dispenser

These items can make life easier and more comfortable, and they are available in local stores at reasonable prices. Most can be installed by you or by a family member. A vanity chair or stool to sit on is also a welcome amenity in the bathroom.

Taking a bath or a shower can, without a doubt, be unnerving. Some homes have both a bathtub and a separate shower stall. Use both safely with the following adjustments. First, there should be a sufficient amount of easy-to-install anti-slip strips on both surfaces to prevent slipping, unlike the suction cup bathmat that tends to attract mould and mildew and must be removed regularly and sanitized.

Both the bathtub and the shower area should have a water-appropriate small chair, seat, or board to sit comfortably and safely. An adjustable shower column with a handheld showerhead with a long flexible hose will be highly beneficial. Include a wall-mounted soap dispenser. Corner caddies are helpful to hold amenities. For a shower stall, a telescopic adjustable shower caddy in the appropriate location to have the required amenities also provides a safe way to store what you need during a bath or shower—even while sitting down—with conveniently situated hooks and accessible bars for hanging clothing and towels.

Enhance safety getting in and out of a bathtub and a shower stall by using strategically placed grab bars. These must be well anchored on solid wood studs behind walls. For a shower within the bathtub, install a sturdy bath rail or tub grip on the raised side of the tub to make entering and exiting safer.

If so inclined, you can consider transforming your current bathtub into one of several options. The first two options transform your bathtub into a shower stall type with a varying entry height of the finished changeover, which, unfortunately, eliminates the possibility of taking a bath. Other options will transform the tub into a shower stall with the convenience of a watertight door for taking a bath. Follow the link to visualize options.[28]

Various devices can help take a mobility-restricted person into a bathtub. Any one of these options requires an investment. Should you plan to renovate the bathroom, the marketplace has several options to choose from that would probably meet your needs. However, removing and installing new bathroom fixtures does require removing all previous fixtures, a project that will require a reputable and reliable contractor.

Some shower stalls or bathtubs do not have proper lighting, though they might have a fan to expel humidity.

If so, consider replacing it with a model with both a fan and a light. If neither is available, consider placing a dehumidifier to remove the humidity, thus limiting mildew.

To increase illumination while in the bathtub or shower, think about using the type of shower curtain often seen in hotels instead of the standard privacy curtain. The top 25 to 30 percent of the curtain is either sheer or see-through vinyl, which lets ambient light in, while the lower part is opaque, which for some models, snaps on and off for easy washing. This option provides privacy yet more light and safety inside the bathtub or shower stall.

Handheld electrical items, such as hairdryer, hair clipper, and all other electrical devices, should be unplugged and stored away when not in use. When in use, keep away from the sink or the bathtub, especially when filled with water.

As discussed in prior sections, proper lighting is critical in the bathroom. Switches must be easily accessible. Install motion sensor lights or nightlights in corridors and the bathroom.

CHAPTER 16

Laundry Room / Utility or Storage Room / Garage

Now that I have covered the home's main areas, there remain possible other rooms or spaces that you may or may not frequently visit; however, they also need attention and possible reorganization. Regardless of your frequency of use, good lighting is critical and accessible upon entry. Passageways should be as wide as possible and free of obstructions of any kind. As mentioned earlier, it should have smoke and carbon monoxide detectors.

The laundry area is often a small space. It would be advantageous to separate your laundry by type before entering that area. If there is more space, it could be done directly in that area, maybe on a small table or with shelving for storing the various products in an easily accessible location. If space is limited, the marketplace now offers different cleaning products that require minimal space. They are like strips of paper that dissolve and wash your clothes and a similar one to put in the dryer.[29] Using "green" bleach will eliminate errors in the quantity used when using such a product. A small chair to sit on also makes that task easier to complete.

> During the work completed to construct a full bathroom on the main floor to increase ease of use upon returning from the barn, my mother convinced my father to transform part of the vast kitchen area into a laundry area, which had lots of cupboard space. The kitchen table was the sorting area. This configuration became even more helpful in later years. During the first ten years I cared for my mother, and when I came every other weekend to give Denise some time off, I brought my laundry to do while still chatting with my mother.

The utility or storage area is typically the home of the hot water tank, heating and air conditioning system, and rarely used items, such as suitcases, sporting or exercise equipment, etc. Again, proper lighting is crucial, and the area may be equipped with reliable shelving for stored items such as non-perishables and perishables (with a piece of white tape with the expiry date), especially when the kitchen does not have a pantry; closet space to store seasonal clothing; sometimes a secondary freezer; and other items.

Stored items should be easily accessible on sturdy shelving units, hopefully without having to double up items on top of each other, ensuring that frequently used things are at the appropriate height and that the weights of individual items are within your capacity to handle comfortably.

It is not unusual to find perishables that have gone past the expiry date or dried up, such as in the case of paints and solvents. Regular review of what one would find in the storage area allows one to discard unhealthy food items. Take the opportunity to give away things you no longer have a use for, however, might be of use to someone else. Most cities offer one or more dates to bring dangerous and toxic products to the appropriate location to be safely discarded or recycled.

These suggestions also apply to the garage. Sometimes, the garage can store things such as unused furniture, out-dated television sets, worn tires, no longer usable construction materials from a previous renovation or repair, and much more, to the point where there is no room to put a car during the colder season. With family members' and friends' help, these areas will be made safer. They will find ways to store the items you still need, and all those deemed no longer needed, can be earmarked to sell during a yard sale, given to family and friends, or transported to a recycling station for people in need via local charities.

An organized garage facilitates putting the car inside during colder seasons and eliminating snow removal before an outing. As discussed earlier, if you have retained snow removal services, the driveway must be kept clear. You might also consider having the entrance sidewalk and steps cleaned if you find this task too challenging. If not, you can use a lightweight shovel located either inside the vestibule or readily accessible in the garage to maintain a safe environment for you and your loved ones. Having a garage door opener from within the car can also make the process easier to manage.

In the following chapters, I share ideas and things to consider when relocating. Including the different aspects and situations seniors might want to consider during such a move, such as moving to a smaller home that better meets your needs, moving in with a welcoming family member, moving in with close friends in a similar situation, or moving to a retirement home.

Instructions to complete the interior checklist:

- Using the complete interior checklist in Appendix V, review each area descriptor to determine if it is risk-free of falls or any other dangerous situation. A completed sample follows.

- If the area is safe, write OK or put a ✓, then move to the next item. If useful, there is space to add other descriptors.

- If a precarious situation is identified, then decide what action you intend to take, who will support you in taking action, and when required, identify a contractor or a supplier.

Sample Interior Checklist – Eliminating/
Minimizing Risks of Mishaps

Risk Free	Description of Area	Action to Take	Support from Family and Friends	Investigate Probable Contractor
✓	Proper lighting			
	Anti-slip strips or secured rugs	Buy/install		
	Kitchen D-style handles	Buy/install	Neighbour	
	Appropriate small appliances			Research
OK	Smoke/ Carbon monoxide detectors			
	Etc.			

Throughout the chapters in Part 5, 'Interior Environment,' there are a number of suggestions of items, devices, and accessories that you may have read about and found useful to purchase or take out of storage, as a means of improving your day-to-day activities. In Appendix VI, I have provided you with a tool titled, 'Checklist of Items to Enhance Quality of Life,' to keep track of such items, especially in seeking out specials or discounted prices. I certainly encourage you to identify current pricing and to keep an eye for sales, to save a few dollars, rather then buying these in one fell swoop.

The following is an example of how this tool could be utilized.

Sample Checklist – Items to Enhance Quality of Life

Item For ... Area	Quantity	Regular $	$ Sale At:
Raised toilet seat	2	$50 – 70*	TBD**
Grab bars for bathtub/ shower stall[30]	6		
Toilet grab bar	2	$35 –140*	
Etc.			

* Depending on chosen style and supplier

** TBD = to be determined

PART 6
Staying or Moving?

Reading about all these possible adjustments or changes in the previous chapters might be daunting. First, decide what you want to do. Do you want to remain in your home for as long as possible? Are your needs being met in your current location? Do you want to downsize to something smaller? Have you been invited to come and live with a family member or close friend? Would you be comfortable sharing your home with a vetted stranger such as a student, nurse, or close friend who would appreciate a lower rent in exchange for helping you out? Or do you want to move to a retirement home?[31]

Once you have arrived at a pretty good idea of what you would like to do, then discuss with your children the challenges you are currently experiencing and how, from your perspective, you think most of these might be remedied by proceeding with your idea.

Research shows beyond any doubt that seniors first and foremost wish to remain in the home of their choice. You want your children and other family members to understand and determine how they can help you achieve this goal. It's also probably not a good idea to start this during the cold season unless there are mitigating factors.

Suppose you decide to continue living in your current home or move to one of the above options. In such cases, the activity of adjusting your environment or rightsizing will still require your focus and that of family and friends. Instead of trying to do everything, focus on one room, probably the kitchen or your bedroom. Work your way at it over several weeks, making a list of items that are no longer needed.

If you have a garage or space that can accommodate excess furniture or other items, then put them there for the time being. Once several rooms are rearranged and adjusted to your needs, share the list with family members, friends, and neighbours, inviting interest to acquire/purchase, which will liberate the temporary staging area for the next room. Offer stuff that remains to various charitable organizations, such as Habitat for Humanity.

The sheer thought of moving away from where you have lived for so many years can be pretty overwhelming. Many emotions and challenges can surface. Such feelings are normal and familiar to most.

> Mother lived in her home on the farm for fifty years. She took some ten years from the time I started talking about moving in with me to decide to accept my offer. Though I implemented everything possible to make her life comfortable, the height of ceilings made it very challenging to maintain sufficient heat during the colder months, which was too much over time. So she processed it and made a choice.

Upon completing the various tools in earlier chapters (Appendixes I, II, and III), you may have concluded that staying in your current home might not be realistic. Even after considering and possibly implementing many of the suggested changes and adjustments, the answer might be that you can no longer remain in your current environment.

There are several factors to contemplate during the assessment and decision-making process. The first factor is the financial investment, including personal investment and the effort required to arrive at viable solutions to transform the current environment into a senior-friendly home. You also have explored various mortgage tools available in the marketplace. Follow the link to the Canada Mortgage and Housing Corporation for information.[32]

A second factor is the amount of energy and personal time you must invest in the regular maintenance and upkeep of the house, especially when it involves numerous steps between basement laundry rooms, the kitchen and living room, and bedrooms and bathroom on upper floors.

A third factor is transportation options. Travelling by car may have become difficult, and public transit may not be readily accessible or available.

CHAPTER 17

What Next?

Consider the result of your 'Likes and Dislikes' assessment in Chapter 6 (Appendix I) when choosing to move to a smaller residence. Furthermore, take a look at the factors described below to spark your thinking and reflection during your analysis, not ignoring all other particular aspects that pertain to your circumstances.

Investment, time, and energy required for a viable solution

Making structural and significant adjustments can be costly and possibly not feasible, things like:

- Building an add-on room
- Building a second full bathroom
- Installing a stair lift because of a narrow staircase, or a tubular elevator due to the absence of space is expensive and sometimes not possible due to certain limitations

- Obtaining building permits can be challenging due to local zoning laws, especially when it may be an encroachment on neighbours

- Should you consider one of the many mortgage-related products? They can be helpful depending on your circumstances. Nonetheless, do so wisely, as they tend to come with accumulated and compounded interests collected at the sale of the house. Always take the required time to weigh the pros and cons and resist any pressure to agree to something that intuitively does not feel right.

Maintenance and upkeep of the house

Your current home was probably the one you chose to fit your needs and a growing family in years past. In most situations, your children have grown up into independent adults with families of their own, though occasionally visiting. Moreover, maintaining a large house is demanding and, depending on circumstances, can be formidable.

About a year after my mother passed away, I found that our small bungalow had become more imposing than life, a perception I experienced due to the emptiness, silence, and solitude. I lacked the motivation and energy to do some of the basic tasks and chores. Instead, I threw myself at my work and rebuilding my relationships with friends that I, unfortunately, put on the back burner while caring for my mother—challenging at best. I decided to sell the house and move to something smaller, closer to my work and friends.

Driving challenges

Unfortunately, when a senior loses their lifelong partner, regrettably, they often turn out to be the sole driver of the household. Sadly, when one or both partners' driving ability and capacity diminishes, their means of getting to and from different locations for appointments, shopping, or personal travel are jeopardized significantly.

Reducing freedom and mobility can be taxing, especially when there is no apparent replacement, such as public transit. We all wish to be as independent as possible in our day-to-day lives, regardless of our age. Being cut off from that autonomy is stressful and, to a certain degree, quite disturbing.

> After spending several months in the hospital fol-
> lowing her illness in 1982, my mother, still in a frail
> condition, went back to her adjusted and reorganized
> home on the farm. She certainly could not drive,
> and to make matters worse, her eyesight slowly
> diminished over the following couple of years, which
> unfortunately eliminated any possibility of ever using
> her car again.

Remoteness of children, grandchildren, and service providers

Often, children have become more mobile than we might have been, and their careers may have brought them to a distant location that, regrettably, limits or reduces family visits. The area of your current home may be far from the various service providers and the amenities you appreciate. In years past, you may have been travelling back and forth to work so you could easily pick up the items you needed. However, these long drives to see family or to do some shopping may have become a bit too much.

Seven years before I retired, I purchased my current home, 190 km (118 miles) return from my work. It was an intentional decision as I longed to get back to the quietness and tranquillity of a rural area. At the time, travelling back and forth to work was no big deal. However, as my retirement neared, the two hours a day drive and the increasing speeding of drivers became quite stressful, tiring, and on many occasions dangerous, not ignoring the financial burden of the increasing costs of gasoline and wear and tear on my car.

To support you in conducting a final review of your choice to move to a smaller residence, along with aiding with selecting a different place to settle down, check out at the end of this chapter, the sample assessment, "Decision-Making Factors." Appendix VII has a blank version.

I have listed four dominant factors, though you may have others, depending on your particular circumstance, including the various aspects to ponder during your decision-making process. For each, enter the information that pertains to your situation. Be sure to correlate with the result of your 'Likes and Dislikes' assessment. Based on all the available information that has brought you to a residence that better meets your needs and expectations, doing so in or near your current area might be the answer.

Such a move maintains familiarity with the neighbourhood and accessibility to the desired amenities such as groceries, banking, doctors, car maintenance or public transit, pharmacy, etc. Furthermore, proximity to friends and possibly some family members make moving into a smaller home or a condo or simply renting an apartment increases the attractiveness of such a decision.

However, should your current location no longer meet your needs and expectations, the following section highlights critical elements to appraise and contemplate before making your final decision. Regardless of one's choice, it is crucial to explore the areas of interest for the availability of the various service providers mentioned previously.

Closely examine the following:

- The first thing is to visit areas of interest during the day and the late evening. Certain things happen only during the day while others only during the evenings, sometimes all night.

Years ago, I rented an apartment in a Montreal suburb. I liked it; the price was affordable, so I signed a lease. A few weeks later, I moved in. A few days later, after going to bed, I was awakened by a deafening noise. I got up and went to the bedroom window and discovered that I was directly in line with one of the airport runways used for arrivals and departures. That night, the wind direction set everything up to make the loudest noise—perfectly aligned above my apartment.

- Observe the impact of streetlights and the illumination level. Blinding nightlights might hinder a good night's sleep. You might be near an area with loud noises due to manufacturing, airport, transit system garage, entertainment and bars, railway crossings, sports venues, etc.

- Are you within a reasonable walking distance or a short public transport ride from the services and amenities you enjoy?

- How far are you from family and friends?

- Would an early summer sunrise impact the bedroom and your sleep? Maybe you're an early riser; hence, you would enjoy that aspect. Where does it set? Sunsets are usually spectacular.

- Is there a reasonable size veranda or balcony for you to sit and enjoy sunsets or sunrises? Is there room for a few planters for your favourite vegetable and herbs? If looking at apartments or condos, is there secure entry and exit, or is there a concierge on duty at all times?

- How about accessibility? Elevator or stairs, steps or gradual walkway? Roof deck or outside garden area?

- Is there access to a reliable public transit system? You might not need to have a car or at least not have to use it very often. Suppose you keep your vehicle to enhance your mobility options. When looking for a small bungalow, is secure parking available, regardless if it is in a condo or apartment building sub-basement or a garage?

Go back to your list of 'Likes and Dislikes' to determine that you can satisfy as many 'Likes' as you possibly can and now have to experience the negative aspects of your 'Dislikes.' Please do not leave anything to chance, nor should you make unvalidated assumptions, assertions, or statements as they could turn out as a source of disappointment in the future.

Instruction to complete the assessment, 'Decision-Making Factors':

- Start with columns two, three, and four, going down to each row to capture the appropriate information. The grey areas tend not to apply to this tool. See the following example for clarification.

- Write in your cost (or a contractor's cost, if you use one) to complete two, three, and four. In the example, the contractor's fee is for landscaping duties.

- For the following row, insert the time it takes you to complete these activities.

- In the next row, write down the energy (low to high) you need to exert to complete the tasks.

- The 'Capability and Capacity' row represents the level of challenge (easy to difficult) required to complete the activity.

- The next row deals with travel time with public transit (availability and cost) for your convenience and the convenience of seeing family.

- The following row deals with the services and amenities you require and use, as well as the distance you travel to see family and friends.

- The last row pertains to your family's cost to come and see you.

- After completing columns two, three, and four, <u>go back to column one</u>. This would be useful when you are researching the possibility of conducting renovations to make you environment conducive to your expectations.

- For each project, enter the projected costs.
- For major projects (with or without building permits), such as a stair lift instead of a bathroom on main floor, enter the cost.
- Enter the expected time required to make these improvements.
- Then in the following columns, enter as you have in columns two, three, and four, the energy required of you for these projects and the level of challenge exerted on you.

This type of information should help you in your decision-making process.

Sample – Decision Making Factors

1) Structural Improvements	2) Ongoing Maintenance	3) Local Travel Challenges	4) Travel to and from Family
Costs for Projects **a) Other bathroom – $8500** **b) Railing for entrances – $3200**	Cost for You or Contractors	Your Travel Cost	
	Landscaping $1250	Monthly Pass $80	Gas, etc. $250
Building Permits **Check zoning by-law**			
Space Availability **Stair lift - $3700**			
Plumbing/Electrical **Included above**			
Contractor Time	Your Time to Complete *		
5-7 months	**Inside – 10-15 hrs. monthly**	30 min./trip	4-5 hrs. quarterly
Energy Required from You **			
1-2	3	2	4-5
Capability and Capacity to Complete **			
	3-4	2-3	3-4

			Public Transit **Close by**	Public Transit **None**
			Services' Proximity **Yes**	Distance to Travel **325 km**
				Family Member's cost **$250**

Correlate with 'Likes and Dislikes' – Calculate and enter the cost to assess the investment.

* Amount of hours required for completing.

** Needed personal energy/challenge:

1 = very low, 2 = low, 3 = average, 4 = high, 5 = very high

Note: Grey areas may be not applicable

CHAPTER 18

Suggestions and Tips During the Downsizing Process

Once you have a pretty good idea of the type of smaller dwelling you intend to move into, you will undoubtedly have to part with many items such as furniture, decorative items, and so on, many having fond memories and stories. When it comes to decorative items such as original artwork and antique furniture, consider seeking out the going value with professionals. Sometimes, some pieces that have been in the family for generations might be priceless.

Alas, to follow their dreams and career, the younger generations tends to have a far more mobile and minimalistic lifestyle than the baby boomer generation aspired to during their heydays. Sadly, the level of interest by your children may vary significantly from your perceptions and expectations concerning some of your accumulated loving treasures and memories.

Please don't be offended at their lack of interest. Times are different! Your fancy teacups and saucers, your bulky dining room set, and your cherished mementos are associated with your interests and desires, not necessarily theirs.

Obtaining the room sizes of your next residence will make it easier for planning. The first step is to take the necessary time to identify all the pieces of furniture that you frequently use by putting a strip of masking tape in an inconspicuous area, the green or blue one used by painters, with the anticipated future location, if you know.

When downsizing from a larger home that housed the entire family for many years to a smaller residence, you will probably have to choose what goes and what does not.

When my mother called to accept my offer to move in with me, her chosen arrival timeline provided me with about six months to prepare. Over the summer months, I asked Denise to observe my mother's routine and put pieces of tape on every piece of furniture used consistently, including their location. I purchased a house as our future home, which was smaller than my mother's house.

Access to it a month before my mother's move provided me with the opportunity to establish room sizes and layouts, which made it a bit easier to decide what could be moved and what would have to remain in the farmhouse. I wanted to bring as much of my mother's furniture as possible so she would recognize it and become more comfortable with this significant change in her life.

Some items were added, such as furniture for a spare bedroom, dining room furniture, a secondary sofa, and chairs for my basement living room. Sadly, I was compelled to leave some due to their large sizes. For example, the beautiful rosewood bookshelf cabinet remained in the house. It stood three metres (almost ten feet). Another piece was the massive original painting gifted to my parents many years earlier on their fortieth wedding anniversary.

Wherever you intend to set up your next home, there will be items other than furniture that will require your attention. Moving to a smaller house, a condo, or an apartment, there are tools, clothing, artwork, garden equipment and furniture, and numerous other things that you will probably no longer need or should reduce, given the undoubtedly minimal room to store. Though some buildings include a small storage area, when they are available, they often are the size of a medium closet, hence with minimal space. Reviewing and deciding what you will do with these treasured items will undoubtedly be daunting and no doubt overwhelming. Consider using the 'Downsizing Checklist—Furniture, Accessories, Décor, etc.,' at the end of this chapter.

Other miscellaneous items will also require your attention. Small electric and hand tools might be your starting point, often less emotional unless, of course, you are a consummate handy person. Take your favourite toolbox or get a medium-size one and choose the essential tools you are sure to use in your next home, plus maybe a portable electric drill that will be helpful for some handy work around the house. Next, check with family members to determine their interests.

Hand and garden tools, patio furniture, and garden décor are often relatively easy to sell to people starting their own homes. Older tools and devices can often get some good money from collectors or at a garage sale. A good friend of mine reconditions antique tools. They look great and sell for a reasonable price. This could become your future hobby.

The assessment instrument 'Downsizing Checklist for Miscellaneous Items' should help you determine what you intend to keep and give to family and friends, sold or discarded.

Clothing is often another item that may require your attention when moving to a new home with less storage area and few closets. Generally speaking, it's a good idea to review all of the items in our wardrobe every other year or so and think back if we have actually worn them in the past two or three years.

Seasonal clothing might require reflection on several past seasons to ensure you do not discard garments that you might not wear because of fluctuations in weather. You can donate items that are still in good condition to various charitable organizations for people who would appreciate a warm coat or boots or that pair of pants, shirt, or sweater you wore back in the day but no longer do today.

Another option is to contact a local church or community centre. They might be aware of people who need all sorts of furnishing and accessories after experiencing dramatic and destructive situations.

A few years back, when she was rightsizing, my sister had several excellent pieces of furniture and a double bed to give away. Attempts to sell went unanswered. She contacted her church, and they directed her to a family who had lost almost everything when a tornado hit the region, destroying many dwellings. They picked up everything, and when they offered some money, she declined. They were delighted. There is an old saying (my version): "A person's discarded items is another's treasure." This expression speaks to the reality that things may have contradictory qualities to different people.

Instructions to complete the downsizing checklists:

- The instructions apply to both lists. As indicated earlier, you can identify all the furniture, accessories, décor, etc., with a piece of tape, written with your initial intention of what to do.

- Once labelling is completed, list the items you intend on taking with you and those you probably will not, according to the four categories of the list.

Sometimes you may want to give to family/friends; however, they may decline. Then try to sell it.

- This tool does work best when you know where you are moving. If still an unknown, using a pencil to write information is probably safer until you know more.

Sample Downsizing Checklist— Furniture, Accessories, Décor, etc.

Furniture, Accessories and Decorative Items	Location and Size	Keep and Move	Action		
			Give to Family or Friends	Sell	Give to Charity or Discard
Love seat	Living room 6 X 32"	Yes			
Wide screen TV	Living room 54"	Yes			
Office desk	6' x 40"	No	X	X	
Etc.					

Sample Downsizing Checklist—Miscellaneous Items

Miscellaneous Items	Location	Keep and Move	Action		
			Give to Family or Friends	Sell	Give to Charity or Discard
Band saw	Utility room			X	
Excess tools	Storage room		X	X	X
Wheelbarrow	Shed		X	X	
Etc.					

PART 7

Moving to . . .

Ageing at home provides autonomy, freedom, and independence, facilitating connection to the social network developed over many years. The majority of seniors consider their home as an indicator of social status that is familiar and encompasses fond memories and attachment, while at the same time offering physical and psychological security.

Sadly, numerous factors may require seniors to make a significant and often difficult decision and contemplate an alternative residence or a different perspective. Fortunately, today's mobile seniors with relatively manageable medical ailments may have access to opportunities about when, where, and with whom they might consider living compared to the twentieth century, though sometimes it's not overtly evident. The Canadian landscape has several housing options that befit a range of budgets, health considerations, needs, and individual desires.

Some of the options are as follows:

- Moving in with a welcoming family member, with or without their own family, is often called multigenerational living. Such a decision can be problematic for everyone involved and will undoubtedly include financial and personal costs for all parties. Such an arrangement requires thorough planning.

- Sharing your home with a family member is an inverse take on the preceding option. Often used when the parent has a larger house that can better accommodate everyone. It involves the same caveats and requires reflection and planning.

- Sharing your home, also called co-housing, involves living with one or more close friends and sometimes a vetted stranger. Benefits include cost sharing, companionship, support with tasks, etc. However, this approach may bring about challenges such as privacy.

- Co-operative housing, a type of non-profit housing, is sometimes privately owned or government subsidized. By living in a co-op, you become a member with responsibility for managing the building. You must qualify to access a co-op.[33]

- Supportive housing is open to Canadians whose care needs are not available in their home, nor do they need the level of care provided in a long-term care home, and they cannot afford market rental costs for assisted-living housing.[34]

- Retirement communities tend to have a tiered structure based on the needs of their members, from independent living to semi-dependent living to assisted living.[35]

- Retirement homes, designed for a community of independent and active seniors with access to significant financial support and recreational resources, are for-profit businesses.

- Like retirement homes, the long-term or assisted living facilities are sometimes operated as not-for-profit residences by various government jurisdictions, offering comprehensive health care and support services for seniors with higher care needs.

CHAPTER 19

Multigenerational Living with Family

Moving in with a welcoming family member requires thoughtful consideration, reflection, and communication between yourself and family members. Once there is consensus on the viability of such an arrangement, it also clearly establishes who is moving in with whom. Over the following weeks or months, all parties must further discuss needs and expectations, their definition and clarification, and their acceptance. On occasion, the senior parents move in with an adult child, like my mother, who moved in with me.

In other cases, should the parent still reside in the original family home, it could also permit an adult child and their family to move into the roomier environment. Whether it's a single senior parent or both parents, and whether the adult child has a family of their own or not, such a significant life change will be troubling and challenging for all concerned. Having completed the 'Likes and Dislikes' assessment is an excellent starting point to engage in the conversation that would bring to light benefits and challenges.

Multigenerational living focuses on various elements such as economics, caregiving, mutual support, and other perspectives, such as reducing travel to provide caregiving support, cost control when home care and assisted living costs are out of reach, increasing time together and companionship for a parent to eliminate loneliness, bonding with grandchildren, supporting around the home on basic tasks and activities, and financial assistance. These are often the most common challenges to be addressed.

However, such arrangements are not guaranteed to work. A thorough assessment of the motive for such an arrangement should **not** be rooted in guilt, attempting to fix past parental or childhood issues or seeking to earn a parent's or child's love and respect. A problematic and somewhat tense relationship between parent and adult child is unlikely to improve by moving in with each other. Family living drawbacks may include space issues, time for self, emotionally demanding and stressing expectations, perception of returning to live together, present and future caregiving duties, and practicality.

Here are a few suggested—and essential—conversation points to support you in setting boundaries that ought to occur before any decision:

- Honest and genuine conversations concerning specific needs and expectations, emphasizing dialogue, openness, and compromise on differing views, specifically involving everyone impacted, even though they may not be decision-makers, such as young children

- Defining clear, understood, and agreed to roles and responsibilities

- Accessibility and mobility within the home, such as stairs

- Availability and proximity of some social life or activities

- Space usage: expectations of family life, one bathroom shared by all or two or more bathrooms, competing for television viewing/music listening, access to their own kitchen/meals (i.e., who cooks, mealtimes, family or self, cleaning after meals), house cleaning, laundry, etc.

> With my roommate, if I prepare meals, then he cleans up. If he cooks, then I clean up. In my previous book about our journey—*Lasting Touch*—I shared many examples of what I did to provide as much autonomy to my mother on many aspects of her day-to-day life, which is critical for seniors' dignity.

- Participation or exclusion from the family holiday or events

- Personal cost such as privacy issues linked to work schedule, individual needs such as a quiet area for reflection or downtime, respectful of private space/bedroom

- Financial participation in multigenerational living arrangements will possibly increase utility costs, food requirements due to limitations or diet requirements, requiring some form of financial participation (i.e., how much, when, and how reimbursed)

- Plus, anything else that you feel needs to be discussed

For instance, my mother and I had already talked about financial issues and her monthly participation. We agreed that I would reassess after a five- to six-month period to see if it required a change. Mother's need for warmth, which had been the major challenge that brought her to decide to accept my offer, had resulted in a slightly more expensive issue than anticipated. The house temperature was around 25 to 26° C (low 80s° F) to maintain mom's comfort, though on weekends, you would have seen me in summer clothes all winter. The new agreement changed to have a slight financial increase during the winter season.

Regardless of all the information highlighted, it would probably be helpful and wise to ponder a trial period of three to six months. In some cases, seniors have rented out their house on popular websites during that interval. Such a period would allow everyone to experience this new and very different lifestyle.

You could do an evaluation and review to ascertain the experience and decide if it should become a formal arrangement or take a different direction. Having considered, discussed, and done a bit of research or exploration of next steps or other options, it would also be prudent should the trial period not result in a mutually satisfactory outcome.

I have friends who, upon their retirement, sold all their assets and started travelling to different parts of Canada and other countries, based on their likes and appreciation of winter sports activities. Through it was to be a trial for three years, it has been now over eight years and they are still enjoying the travel, though they probably stayed put somewhere during the pandemic.

CHAPTER 20

Multigenerational Living with Non-family Members

Though this option may not seem realistic and possibly somewhat uncomfortable, it is still a worthy option that merits exploration. Sharing your home with a roommate is not for everyone, as it depends on your circumstances, personality, needs, and values. Many seniors' organizations, churches, and community centres can provide you with information about such an option and often support you in finding several suitable and vetted candidates that you can interview to decide if you wish to engage in such an arrangement.

Seniors who have a spare bedroom or maybe a well-organized basement area, and who are comfortable sharing part of their home, can let their network know they are looking for a live-in helper or can contact a local college or university. On occasion, these institutions have waiting lists of students looking for a room in residence or, due to their finances, are looking for a low-cost room and board option in exchange for helping out around the house.

Many years ago, while in a new job and experiencing difficulty finding a more suitable place to live, a colleague introduced me to her elderly friend's home. She was looking for a person to do various tasks around the house in exchange for a reduced rent. The agreement was beneficial for both of us and lasted several years until I moved away to care for my mother.

Earlier I mentioned that after an unfortunate incident, I decided to make some significant changes to my lifestyle, which I did. About a year later, my friend, who came over some weekends to help with the more demanding tasks, lost his job due to the pandemic and could no longer afford his rent. For several days I reflected on the situation from different angles. I had a spare bedroom in the basement so we both would have our privacy.

We discussed it, and he moved in at the end of the month. He has his quarters, I have mine upstairs, we share the rest of the house, and he helps out with many tasks. The arrangement turned out to be a winning combination for both of us, especially this past winter, which was abundant in the quantity of snow.

Make sure you have a venue to communicate any possible uncomfortable roommate issues or behaviours. Do not tolerate!

This option could be with a friend who is in a relatively similar housing situation. However, before you jump into such a situation, especially when that person's character is somewhat nebulous to you, suggest going on an extended vacation together. Travelling with someone and sharing accommodations for three or four weeks usually identifies one's personality and character and might reveal a possible mutual affinity or not. Regardless, most of the above discussion points remain pertinent, as well as the following benefits and challenges.

Consider the pros and cons of home sharing:

- <u>Quiet versus animated environment:</u> Do you prefer your solitude, or do you long for some ability to interact with others?

- <u>Other housing options:</u> Have you explored other possibilities, such as multigenerational family living or different types of housing options, that might better meet your needs?

- <u>Freedom and independence:</u> Do you prefer self-determination to do what you desire without considering others in the household, or would a trusted roommate's help and support be appreciated?

Support organizations: Research and seek out organizations that can provide you with information and guidance. These resources should also have taken all possible precautions (vetting, background check, etc.) with candidates. Seniors who have acted on this type of arrangement report higher satisfaction when organizations match people and provide support services when needed. Share your intentions with close friends or neighbours, as they may know a trusted person from a different region coming to your area to study, looking for an affordable place to stay in exchange for helping out around the house.

Proceeding with a roommate: Take the time to write down your needs and expectations, boundaries, and rules to discuss with the future live-in person. Here are a few items to consider:

- Whatever financial considerations agreed to should be paid in a timely fashion.

- Using someone else's things without asking. Is food included?

- Communicate, communicate, communicate, no gossiping.

- Bring up minor issues rather than internal resentment.

- If applicable, create a cleaning schedule for specific chores.

- Clean up after yourself.

- Respect personal and shared space.

- If only one bathroom, be respectful of usage.

- When applicable, share cooking.

- Practice the "platinum rule."[36]

- Plus, whatever is essential for you.

Once you have narrowed your search to one or two candidates, if not already done, you can have a background check or you could also ask the potential candidate to get one, just like many employers do with future employees. The RCMP is the only official way to perform a criminal background check on someone in Canada.[37]

CHAPTER 21

Other Housing Options

The other housing options described at the beginning of this part—co-operative housing, supportive housing, retirement communities, retirement homes, and long-term or assisted living facilities—are beyond my purview. I would, however, share what I have heard from others. Future housing options, first and foremost, depend on your financial circumstances, your propensity for active living, and your social-focused personality. Second, it is conditional on the level of health care you require to ensure a quality style of living.

Co-operative housing organizations will accept members mainly due to their limited finances. However, admission to long-term or assistive care is due to the requirement of more demanding health care support.

I strongly encourage you to reflect and ponder your circumstances, including current and potential ensuing ailments and medical conditions, during your assessment of future housing. It is always wise and prudent to take a long view, including family history, the realities versus the myths of ageing.[38]

In North America, between 5 and 7 percent of seniors sixty-five and up are in long-term care or assisted living. A significant majority of older adults are active and productive and consistently learn new skills.

Future housing considerations should be well researched and explored via trusted individuals, known resources, and reputable organizations. Please vet all web findings via respected and known organizations. Unfortunately, much misinformation and fraud exist on the web and through unsolicited phone calls. Speaking to people who have experienced similar situations, explorations, and decisions can, by far, be quite revealing and informative.

PART 8
Miscellaneous Ideas

As you advance in your current or new home, there are other actions you might consider taking. For example, in the business world, the word '*Kaizen*' is a Japanese term meaning change for the better or continuous improvement. "It is a Japanese business philosophy regarding the processes that continuously improve within the workplace." [39]

Analogous to that definition, could we not contemplate associating "the change for the better" concept to our house, home, and lives. But as mentioned earlier, it would mean adhering to the cautionary principles.

Consequently, it is crucial to analyze how current and future issues, obstacles, or challenges could negatively impact our health. A correlation to this perspective would be examining what unpredictable and unforeseen scenarios or events might unfold that would also be detrimental to your health, lifestyle, and environment.

CHAPTER 22

Supplementing Our Senses

Human ageing is associated with a wide range of physiological changes that limit our normal functions and render us more susceptible to particular challenges or inconveniences. These variations ARE NOT necessarily diseases. We all change, as we grow older. Some systems slow down, while others lose the 'fine-tuning.' As a general rule, slight, gradual changes are common, and most of these tend to require us to adapt and be patient with ourselves.

Our senses will experience some form of decline as we age. Though the sense of taste, touch, and smell tend to, over time, deteriorate for many people, regardless of their age, the most noticeable change for seniors is vision and hearing. Unfortunately, it often starts with what seems to be minor shifts that we tend to disregard, equating it to fatigue and sometimes pride.

Visible World

One of these changes is our vision. Because the reduction is gradual, we tend to instinctively adapt and postpone getting it checked. Unfortunately, there could be a more severe condition lurking below the surface.

> Though my mother was diagnosed with tunnel vision, her doctor never explored what might be the cause. After the dramatic discovery of her diabetes, I wondered if her limited eyesight had suffered the same disregarded fate. A visit to an ophthalmologist confirmed my suspicion. Mother had cataracts in both her eyes. After undergoing the procedure, Mother got between 25 and 35 percent of her eyesight back, giving her the ability to read large font books and watch television.

That incident led me to conclude that a second or third opinion, vis-à-vis a medical concern, would be my approach in the future.

Though I have previously highlighted the importance of ensuring appropriate lighting in all areas of your house, sometimes improving the wattage will often enhance the luminosity of an otherwise dimly lit room. However, other situations will require additional lighting with floor or table lamps and clip lamps. When not possible, incorporating timers, motion-sensing lights, or chargeable nightlights in most rooms will increase safety.

Use different colours to contrast specific rooms, such as kitchen counters versus kitchenware, a colourful tissue box on top of a white toilet, colourful towels, a bright bedspread, reflector tape to mark edges of stairs and thresholds between rooms, etc.

For convenient and trouble-free access, always place keys and other essential items you tend to take with you when you leave the house in the exact same location. (Note: If using a car fob (wireless key system) to lock your vehicle, never use it to lock your car when there might be someone nearby as they can hack the signal and remove the content or steal the car.)

The same routine applies to eyeglasses, remotes, kitchenware and utensils, and other frequently used items, making them easy to find.

Operating dials of household appliances (stove, dishwasher, washer, dryer, remotes, etc.) often become worn from years of use. To remedy that issue, use contrasting nail polish to mark the OFF indicator.

In my first book, I talked about an incident with my mother, who inadvertently turned on all four stovetop heating elements in her attempt to make some soup while I was away on business. In my mind's-eye, I saw my mother crying. I immediately called to inquire. She was indeed crying and was very agitated, as she could not figure out how to resolve the situation, given her limited vision. What ensued over the following hour describes all the potentially dangerous situations while operating a stove. Hence, my suggestions and tips concerning a stove would significantly be beneficial in minimizing injury.

Audible World

"Hearing loss is the second most prevalent chronic disability among older adults. 20 percent of adults over sixty-five, 40 percent over seventy-five and 80 percent of nursing home residents have a significant hearing problem."[40] A diagnosis of dementia for people with hearing loss can occur, exacerbating possible existing cognitive challenges.

If someone in the household is experiencing hearing challenges, I suggested auditory and visual triggers to alert the home's occupant of a situation requiring their attention in a previous chapter.

Additionally, being in the same well-lit room and facing each other will facilitate communication and understanding. Please make all attempts at speaking and enunciating clearly, not too loud or too soft. Background noises such as a radio, a television, and so on should be either turned down or off when possible.

> My mother's hearing was undoubtedly not an issue for her. I described a hilarious story about that in *Lasting Touch*. During one of several evening outings, she mentioned hearing me driving away going out after she had gone to bed and asked if I had a nice time. I was shocked. After a bit of denial on my part, she exclaimed, "I may be blind, but I'm not deaf." It would seem that she had on countless occasions, heard me drive away.

The technology of hearing aids has improved dramatically. Please seek out the appropriate support from a recognized service provider. Digital technology is far superior to the analogue type of years past.

Gustatory World

We are born with thousands of taste buds located mainly on the tongue. Various circumstances affect how we discern taste, including bacterial infections, nervous system disorders, nutrient deficiencies, nerve damage found along the pathway from the mouth to the brain, several types of medication, smoking, and ageing. Seniors tend to maintain the ability to detect sweet tastes; however, determining sour, salty, and bitter flavours can be challenging.

Regrettably, some seniors will sometimes compensate for the diminishing savours by applying copious amounts of salt on their food, which by all accounts, is not suitable for them and might lead to chronic diseases.

> During the years my mother lived with me, I quickly noticed that unusual behaviour, as I could not recall a high salt usage during meals growing up, except, of course, for the corn on the cob season.

I researched the topic and raised the issue during a meal. Mother's reaction started with a bit of resistance, followed by a maybe, for certain foods. I started looking for a gentle way out and discovered that the marketplace offered various products of dried herbs with no or minimal salt added.

Today, more of these products are available. To enjoy several varieties of flavours and spiciness, I use a product called Mrs. Dash.[41] They have several seasonings, some exotic, which increase the taste level without the unfortunate negative impact of excess salt.

Olfactory World

As we age, our ability to detect and recognize odours tends to decrease, which is also impacted by smoking and some medication. This reduction in smells reinforces the importance of having detectors that alert you when it senses the presence of smoke, carbon monoxide, and other dangerous gases in various parts of the house. Sadly, there is a potential for other odours that can be embarrassing when not noticed.

> Several months after Mother moved in with me, the caregiver brought to my attention—via a short note left in my bedroom —that my mother might be experiencing a light bladder leakage, which might be embarrassing for her if noticed. She suggested a simple solution and even provided a picture of a product for me to purchase. She showed me how to apply one of these pads to each pair of her undergarments. Mother's dignity saved! Nothing gained in mentioning it.

Tactile World

Our skin changes and becomes less flexible as we age. The sensitivity to cold and hot water temperature reduces. Tasks that use motor skills, like picking something up off the floor, opening a jar, removing product wrapping, or manoeuvring pots and pans, may be challenging. Our joints become stiffer, and we might lose some muscle mass as well as our flexibility.

Earlier suggestions intend to make daily life easier and more comfortable, most importantly, reducing the temperature of the hot water system.

Furthermore, if someone in the household struggles with walking because of poor balance or challenges in getting around, explore mobility aids for which there is a wide variety of styles, depending on circumstances and challenges. Another option is to install grab rails in some specific areas of the house. When a wheelchair is required, all passageways must be the appropriate width and obstruction-free to facilitate mobility.

CHAPTER 23

Safety of Parents Versus Parents' Autonomy

Seniors will undoubtedly experience increased attention and possibly a high level of insistence from their children vis-à-vis welfare and safety, especially when the direct contact is sporadic because of their geographic location or busy lives. Another possible situation is that maybe, just maybe, you may not have kept them informed and up to date on what's happening in your life because you don't want to be a burden. You may be experiencing minor issues and ailments, and you no longer are running marathons; however, you consider yourself in good spirits and good health.

Your offspring probably have a fully engaged life, with a family of their own, careers, responsibilities, demands, and pressures. As a result, it is not uncommon for children to suddenly notice and realize that you are no longer the energetic and upbeat parent they remember. Children need to understand their parent's situation and needs better; however, though they probably should figure it out, sometimes they need a parent's guidance.

Sometimes, they might base their conclusions on an unscheduled Zoom call, on the day you chose to spend the day in your jammies, or they show up on your doorstep for a surprise visit while you are lounging enjoying a late morning coffee or tea. It's almost as if, from your children's perspective, overnight, you have aged, and they now must step in to protect you. Expect such a scenario to occur. So, what are you going to do?

From your perspective, yes, you have aged; however, you are still active, in relatively good health, happy to be in your home, and enjoying life to the fullest. You could shut down, refuse to discuss it, and change the subject. Unfortunately, that approach will not help reassure your well-intentioned children nor make such a conversation go away.

A more fruitful approach would be to discuss it in a relaxed setting, like a nice meal, or sitting comfortably in your living room over the beverage of choice, with no one else from the extended family. Such a conversation should not have outside influences or input that could feel like ganging up on you.

Acknowledge that, yes, things are different; however, you are aware of your limitations, and you do not deny them. Share the great things you have been doing and some of the challenges and adjustments you have implemented based on your 'Likes and Dislikes' assessment. Maybe even share a copy. Emphasize how you are enjoying your autonomy and ability to maintain a satisfactory level of control.

Then share the different community support services you occasionally use to make things easier, as well as your activities to keep healthy and connected. In addition, it might be helpful for your children to understand your perspective fully. Your children will undoubtedly respect the opportunity to appreciate your concerns and fears.

> You will remember the story I shared with you about my sister breaking her leg. During the same conversation, she proactively shared that she and her husband abandoned the annual tradition of having an extensive vegetable garden in their backyard, instead planting only potatoes. At the same time, she struck an arrangement with her neighbour who lives alone, who would take on the weeding of the flowerbeds and the potato garden in exchange for my sister doing some small sewing projects, a bit of socializing, and an occasional meal.

As parents, you may have some internal fears and concerns about your age, about leaving your home, or even about going a long-term care or retirement facility. During my interactions with seniors, here are a few of the situations[42] they shared with me:

- Not being capable of living in their own home
- Safety and security issues
- Being unable to manage change
- Unable to drive
- Not being able to maintain a level of control and autonomy over their affairs
- Being rejected or abandoned by family or removed from the familiar surroundings of friends and family

Initiating regular conversations, whether face-to-face or via technology, should put your mind at ease. Plan follow-up conversations, as there are many subjects to put on the table.

As highlighted earlier, one challenging and uncomfortable discussion would address future health issues that might lead to a different living arrangement. Maybe discussing your intention to complete an advanced care planning (ACP)[43] (check out the video that explains ACP[44]), estate and asset planning, and so on would certainly be appropriate.

To fulfill your wishes to be carried out, make them known, often in an official format such as a will. Estate planning was never an easy thing to do. Going forward, being prepared and organized will save your families unwanted headaches and costs. The following site is for sure a great beginning.[45]

Seek out your children's support in respecting your intentions, for the time being anyway. Be aware that emotions often trump logical and rational perspectives. These conversations might at times become animated and even intense. If that should happen, call for a time-out.

Challenged feelings, expectations, and views produce stress hormones that increase our heartbeat, resulting in various levels of anger. Unfortunately, at the same time, judgment seems to decrease substantially. Should you observe an increase of agitation in yourself or others, it is time to call for time out—generally, an hour or more to provide everyone the time to regain their composure.

The following articles should facilitate positive and fruitful conversations:

- "Should safety take priority over independence of older parents?"[46]
- "How to have difficult conversations with your aging parents"[47]

CHAPTER 24

ICE (In Case of Emergency)

Due to unforeseen incidents or emergencies, it is critical to plan all eventualities. Moreover, during a chaotic situation, our focus may not be at its best; thus, we may not have the foresight to act or behave most optimally. Hence, having a fire escape route, a regroup area, and a means of providing valuable information in case of an emergency is vital.

Quick Access to Contacts

In the chapter dealing with the interior of your house, I suggested that you pre-program phone numbers. While in the throes of an emergency, we may not remember numbers and your address. The word "emergency" or "911" or the name of your child makes it much easier to press the button.

Vial of Life

Having your pertinent health information easily accessible by emergency and medical respondents is especially vital in a critical and chaotic situation. It is advisable that you have at minimum, the basic information in your wallet or purse with your identification. It should also include contact information for family members, doctors, specialists, etc.

Additionally, you could also put similar information on your smart phone in the contact section under the word 'ICE.' Savvy emergency personnel could go to your contacts and look for the name 'ICE' and contact information of the person you would like to be notified in an emergency.

It is also a good idea to write all your relevant information and store it in a container, preferably a metal container with a lid labelled "VIAL OF LIFE," keeping it in a readily accessible place like the refrigerator. Do not forget to put a note in **large caps** on the door saying "VIAL OF LIFE" or LIFE (Life-saving Information For Emergencies). Please remember to keep the information up to date.

The customary information generally found in the vial of life is as follows:

- Name, address, gender, phone number, and date of birth of people in the household
- Identifying information, including a picture and description of the person(s)
- Primary language
- Emergency contact names and phone numbers
- Doctor's name, phone number, and possibly, preferred hospital
- Health information such as:
  - Health card number and province of origin
  - Height and weight
  - Past surgeries and hospital circumstances
  - Physical challenges
  - Medical conditions or injuries and allergies
  - Blood type
  - List of medications including non-prescribed
  - Dietary requirements
  - Health insurance information
  - Do not resuscitate order, health care proxy, living wills with appropriate legal documentation
- Plus any information that is required to maintain your safety

You can search on the web to find samples or templates.

PART 9
Conclusion

At this point in the book, you may be feeling somewhat overwhelmed. I agree with you! It's a lot of information to take in. Some suggestions might fit with your needs, and some might not. As indicated previously, I based these ideas and suggestions on my experience as a caregiver and newly discovered information and resources, which were not readily available in the 1980s and 1990s.

For you, the next step is to take some time to digest all this information and decide what works for you, what is exciting information for the future, and what you will ignore or further reflect, for now at least.

I wanted to share what transpired during my fourteen years as a caregiver to my mother, coupled with experiences of good friends who followed in my steps with their parents and loved ones, seniors I had the good fortune to meet and interact with, and my personal experiences about ageing. With this perspective in mind, I shared stories and situations linked to some of these ideas to come alive for you, the reader.

You may have noticed that I have not been very kind toward leaders and governments during these challenging months of the COVID-19 pandemic. However, I believe the implementation of a structural change in the Canadian health care system must take place. It requires a more efficient approach, adapted to the needs of today's citizens and not those of the mid-1950s.

A superior infrastructure based on new and emerging technologies, innovative and creative approaches and processes, best practices from other jurisdictions, competent and savvy leadership, and sound management practices are needed. The twenty-first century is upon us, and it is time to take all Canadians' health seriously. Forming committees to review and analyze is over. In my experience in the business world, a popular definition of a committee is a dead-end street where good ideas and solutions are lured to die. The time for talking is over. Now is the time to act.

The evidence is all around us. Home care for citizens of all ages when not experiencing acute health issues has been successfully demonstrated in many countries, while also reducing overall health-related costs.

Denmark's approach is one of the gold standards. (See endnotes #14 and #15.)

I do not know what the future holds for Canadians and the world senior population. The pandemic has clearly shown the importance of being ready for all eventualities. COVID-19 is not the first pandemic, nor will it be the last. As I write this book, the country is already well in a fourth wave, with more victims paying the price with their lives. Will all the human loss be for nothing?

Regrettably, my generation and older will probably not have the opportunity to experience meaningful change within the health system. Ideally, there is still hope for future generations should world leaders and large corporations stop bickering and stop destroying the planet.

As I write my final words on this second journey, I am grateful to my mother for raising a child who cares for others. My first memoir—*Lasting Touch*—was our story as we journeyed together for nearly fourteen years. My sole goal was to influence more male family members to step up to care for their elders. I believe I have succeeded in doing so.

For this second book, my sole purpose is to provide information that can help seniors remain in the home of THEIR choice for as long they can. Whether this book supports a dozen or a thousand elderly parent in experiencing a safe and quality long-life supported by their children, I will have succeeded.

The well-known saying, "It takes a village to raise a child," can easily be repurposed by stating it as, "It takes a global village to care for our elders."

RESOURCES

- Canada Mortgage and Housing Corporations (CMHC)
  – Maintaining seniors independence through home adaptation – A self-assessment guide: https://www.cmhc-schl.gc.ca/en/professionals/industry-innovation-and-leadership/industry-expertise/senior-housing/maintaining-seniors-independence-through-home-adaptations-a

- Government of Canada – Public Health Agency of Canada (PHAC) – You can prevent falls: https://www.canada.ca/en/public-health/services/health-promotion/aging-seniors/publications/publications-general-public/you-prevent-falls.html

- Government of Canada – Public Health Agency of Canada (PHAC) – A guide to home safety for seniors: https://www.canada.ca/en/public-health/services/health-promotion/aging-seniors/publications/publications-general-public/safe-living-guide-a-guide-home-safety-seniors.html

- McMaster University – Optimal Aging Portal (You can register to receive regular emails on aging): https://www.mcmasteroptimalaging.org

- International Council on Aging – https://www.icaa.cc

- National Council on Aging – https://www.ncoa.org
- Council on Ageing Ottawa (note: chapters in most large cities) – https://coaottawa.ca
- Visavie – Home care support organization in Quebec and Eastern Ontario – https://visavie.com/en/home-care-for-seniors/
- National Institute on Aging (NIA) – Aging in place: Growing older at home https://www.nia.nih.gov/health/aging-place-growing-older-home
- National Institute on Aging (NIA)/Ryerson University – https://www.nia-ryerson.ca/resources
- United Nations - Department of Economic and Social Affairs – Ageing: https://www.un.org/development/desa/ageing/resources-2.html
- Research Institute for Aging (RIA) – https://the-ria.ca
- Age Well, Live Well – Technologies for healthy aging – https://agewell-nce.ca
- Canadian Association for Retired Persons (CARP) – https://www.carp.ca
- Government of British Columbia – https://www2.gov.bc.ca/gov/content/family-social-supports/seniors
- Government of Alberta – https://www.alberta.ca/senior-supports.aspx
- Government of Saskatchewan – https://www.saskatchewan.ca/residents/family-and-social-support/seniors-services

- Government of Manitoba – https://www.gov.mb.ca/seniors/

- Government of Yukon – https://yukon-seniors-and-elders.org

- Government of the Northwest- Territories – https://www.hss.gov.nt.ca/sites/hss/files/seniors_information_handbook.pdf

- Government of Nunavut – https://www.gov.nu.ca/eia/documents/nunavut-seniors-information-handbook

- Government of Ontario – https://www.ontario.ca/page/ministry-seniors-accessibility

- Government of Quebec – https://www.quebec.ca/en/family-and-support-for-individuals/seniors

- Government of Nova Scotia – https://novascotia.ca/seniors/

- Government of New Brunswick – https://www2.gnb.ca/content/gnb/en/departments/social_development/seniors/content/seniors_guide_toservicesandprograms.html

- Government of Prince Edward Island – https://www.princeedwardisland.ca/en/topic/seniors

- Government of Newfoundland & Labrador – https://www.gov.nl.ca/hcs/seniors/

APPENDIX I

Likes and Dislikes Self-Assessment [48]

Likes Appreciated / Convenient	Rate	Dislikes Challenging / Inconvenient	Rate

Total		Total	

Rating: Likes = 1 (low) to 5 (high) Dislikes = -1 (low) to -5 (high)

Note: Use a highlighter pen to identify top 'Likes and Dislikes.'

APPENDIX II

Exterior Checklist – Eliminating/ Minimizing Risks

Risk-Free	Description of Area	I Can Take Action	Support Family & Friends	Investigate Contractor/ Supplier
	Walkways and driveways			
	Proper lighting at entrances			
	Solid stairways, handrails, and porch			
	Anti-slip strips – exterior style			
	Motion sensor lights / Solar lights			
	Bench/table at main entrance			
	Lever style door handles			

Jean-François Pinsonnault

	Peep hole / small window to see outside / storm door screen and lock			
	No-step / no-trip threshold			
	Mailbox access			
	Swing-away hinges for entry (If required)			
	Access ramp for wheelchair (If required)			
	Visible civic address number			
	Branches / trees trimmed			
	Lawn/deck furniture secured			
	Roof and eaves-trough cleaning			
	Exterior window cleaning			
	Landscaping activities			
	Snow removal – driveway			

Snow removal – walkways and staircases			
Minimizing expenses			
Enlisting support			

APPENDIX III

Most-Used Kitchenware, Utensils, Small Appliances

Most-Used Kitchenware, Utensils, Small Appliances, Etc.		
Items	Location	Frequency D = Daily W = Weekly M = Monthly

Jean-François Pinsonnault

APPENDIX IV

Rarely Used Kitchenware, Utensils, Small Appliances

Rarely/Never Used Kitchenware, Utensils, Small Appliances, Etc.		
Items	Location	Next steps SO = Special Occasions G = Give, S = Sell R/T = Recycle/Trash

APPENDIX V

Interior Checklist – Eliminating/ Minimizing Risks

Risk-Free	Description of Area	Action Taken	Support Family and Friends	Investigate Contractor/ Supplier
	Entrance safety			
	Proper lighting			
	Anti-slip strips or secured rugs			
	Deadbolt locks or safety chain			
	Doorbell, visibility, security			
	Lever-style door handle			
	Chair / bench in entrance			
	Closet with proper lighting			

Jean-François Pinsonnault

	Seasonal items stored elsewhere			
	Kitchen / Dining area			
	Proper lighting			
	Motion sensing lights			
	Space to work with chair/stool			
	Frequently used items on convenient shelves			
	Rarely used items elsewhere			
	Kitchen D-style handles			
	Appropriate small appliances			
	Microwave well-located			
	Lazy Susan (if required)			

	Quality "Reacher Grabber"			
	Large appliances (If required)			
	ABC fire extinguishers			
	Anti-slip strips or taped rugs			
	Smaller size containers			
	Lever or touch less faucets			
	Hot water temperature			
	Pet food and water dish			
	Harsh cleaning products			
	Living Room / Bedroom (s)			
	Strategically staged furniture			

	Phones in different areas of the house			
	Pre-programmed phone numbers with large numbers			
	Level thresholds between rooms			
	Anti-slip strips or rugs with double sided tape (all sides)			
	Cords and extensions located along walls			
	Timers on lights			
	Rechargeable nightlights			
	Smoke and carbon dioxide detectors			
	Sturdy side tables			
Bathroom (s)				
	Proper lighting			

Anti-slip strips or rugs			
Convenient fixtures			
Bathtub and shower grab bars			
General bathroom grab bars			
Stored electri-cal devices			
Vanity chair / stool			
Bathtub versus shower stall or both			
Laundry / Storage area			
Appropriate lighting			
Obstacle free passageway			
Sturdy storage shelves and hooks			

	Chair with work table			
Garage			
	Appropriate lighting			
	Sturdy storage shelves and hooks			
	Obstruction-free passageways			
	Accessible light switches or motion-sensor lights			
Other			

Jean-François Pinsonnault

APPENDIX VI

Checklist of Items to Enhance Quality of Life

Item For ... Area	Quantity	Regular $	Sale Price $

Jean-François Pinsonnault

APPENDIX VII

Decision Making Factors

1) Structural Improvements	2) Ongoing Maintenance	3) Local Travel Challenges	4) Travel to and from Family
Costs for Project	Cost for You or Contractor	Your Travel Cost	
Building Permits			
Space Availability			
Plumbing/ Electrical			
Contractor Time	Your Required Time to Complete *		
Energy Required from You **			
Capability and Capacity to Complete **			

		Public Transit	Public Transit
		Services' Proximity	Distance to Travel
			Family Member's Cost

Correlate with "Likes and Dislikes" – Calculate and enter the cost and time to assess the investment.

* Number of hours required for completing.

** Needed energy or challenge:

1 = very low, 2 = low, 3 = average, 4 = high, 5 = very high

Note: Grey areas may be not applicable

APPENDIX VIII

Downsizing Checklist – Furniture, Accessories, etc.

Furniture, Accessories, Decorative Items, Etc.	Location and Size	Keep and Move	Action		
			Give to Family or Friends	Sell	Give to Charity or Discard

APPENDIX IV

Downsizing Checklist – Miscellaneous Items

Miscellaneous Items	Location	Keep and Move	Action		
			Give to Family or Friends	Sell	Give to Charity or Discard

Jean-François Pinsonnault

Sources, Links, Definitions

[1] Source: Sinha, Samir, et al. Bringing Long-Term Care Home: A Proposal to Create a Virtual Long-Term Care @ Home Program to Support a More Cost-Effective and Sustainable Way to Provide Long-Term Care Across Ontario. National Institute on Ageing, November 2020, https://static1.squarespace.com/static/5c2fa7b03917eed9b5a436d8/t/5fd10658e9ed0b03e36cde7b/1607534169740/BringLTCHome_V2.11.17%284%29pdf.pdf. Accessed 23 Aug. 2021.

[2] Source: "Ageing in the Twenty-First Century: A Celebration and A Challenge: Executive Summary," United Nations Population Fund (UNFPA), 2012, https://www.unfpa.org/sites/default/files/pub-pdf/UNFPA-Exec-Summary.pdf. Accessed 23 Aug. 2021.

[3] Source: O'Neill, Aaron, "Life expectancy (from birth) in Canada, from 1800 to 2020," statista, 6 Sep. 2019, https://www.statista.com/statistics/1041135/life-expectancy-canada-all-time/. Accessed 23 Aug. 2021.

[4] According to the World Health Organization, the term *acute care* encompasses a range of clinical health-care functions, including emergency medicine, trauma care, pre-hospital emergency care, acute care surgery, critical care, urgent care and short-term inpatient stabilization. Includes the most time-sensitive, individually oriented diagnostic and curative actions whose primary purpose is to improve health.

[5] According to the World Health Organization, the term *chronic care* is of long duration and generally slow progression. The four

main types … are cardiovascular diseases (like heart attacks and stroke), cancers, chronic respiratory diseases (such as chronic obstructed pulmonary disease and asthma) and diabetes. – Author's note: Over the past decades, various types of dementia have been added to the list.

[6] Source: Feil, Cameron, et al. "Pandemic Perspectives on Long-Term Care: Insights from Canadians in Light of COVID-19," National Institute on Ageing and Canadian Medical Association, 2021, https://static1.squarespace.com/static/5c2fa7b03917eed9b5a436d8/t/60428c8d3c118d6237a6ac11/1614974093703/English+NIA+CMA+Report.pdf. Accessed 23 Aug. 2021.

[7] Source: National Institute on Ageing (NIA) - As COVID-19 exposes a long-term crisis… Page 11 https://www.cbc.ca/news/canada/toronto/covid-ontario-government-home-care-long-term-care-1.5897858 - Accessed 23 Aug. 2021.

[8] Source: Public Broadcasting Service - https://www.pbs.org/show/pbs-fast-forward/ -- YOUTUBE clip: https://www.youtube.com/watch?v=xsDINETTY-8 - Accessed 23 Aug. 2021.

[9] Source: Canadian Institute for Health Information – 1 in 9 new long-term care resident… https://www.cihi.ca/en/1-in-9-new-long-term-care-residents-potentially-could-have-been-cared-for-at-home -Accessed 23 Aug. 2021.

[10] NIA – Bringing Long-Term Care Home - https://static1.squarespace.com/static/5c2fa7b03917eed9b5a436d8/t/5fd10658e9ed0b03e36cde7b/1607534169740/BringLTCHome_V2.11.17%284%29pdf.pdf - Accessed 23 Aug. 2021.

[11] Source: Cautionary Principle – "When an activity raises threats of harm to human health or the environment, precautionary

measures should be taken even if some cause and effect relationships are not fully established scientifically." –https://www.sciencedirect.com/science/article/pii/S0951832018313255 - Accessed 23 Aug. 2021.

[12] Source: Family Caregiving – https://www.helpguide.org/articles/parenting-family/family-caregiving.htm - Accessed 23 Aug. 2021.

[13] Source: The Case of Denmark – https://www.healthcaredenmark.dk/the-case-of-denmark/integrated-care-and-coherence/elderly-care/ - Accessed 23 Aug. 2021.

[14] Source: A Dignified Elderly Care in Denmark - https://www.healthcaredenmark.dk/media/plvbj4yz/elderly-care-v10919.pdf - Accessed 23 Aug. 2021.

[15] Source: Aging Well – https://www.cfn-nce.ca/wp-content/uploads/2021/01/Aging-Well-Queens-Policy-Studies-Final-Report-Master-07.09.2020.pdf - Accessed 23 Aug. 2021.

[16] Source: Aging in Place, Myth or Reality – https://www.rehabmagazine.ca/healthcare/aging-in-place-myth-or-reality/ - Accessed 23 Aug. 2021.

[17] Please include all aspects of one's life – Geographical, Physical, Emotional, and Psychological well-being.

[18] Source: Fall prevention – https://www.canada.ca/en/public-health/services/health-promotion/aging-seniors/publications/publications-general-public/you-prevent-falls.html - Accessed 23 Aug. 2021.

[19] Rona Hardware – Wood stackers - https://www.rona.ca/en/2x4-rack-structure-16-80645098 - Accessed 23 Aug. 2021.

[20] Source: Canada Post on accessibility – https://www.canadapost-postescanada.ca/cpc/en/our-company/about-us/corporate-responsibility/accessibility.page - Accessed 23 Aug. 2021.

[21] Make a list of all the items you no longer wish to keep. Please share it with your family, requesting their level of interest. Next, create a list of whatever is left. Share that with your friends, also asking their level of interest. Finally, whatever items remain, give them to a charity of choice or sell (online or garage sale).

[22] Cloud storage is file storage in the 'cloud'. Instead of keeping your files on your local hard drive, external hard drive, or flash drive, you can save them online. - https://www.lifewire.com/what-is-cloud-storage-2438541 - Accessed 23 Aug. 2021.

[23] Source: Health safety products – https://www.healthcraftproducts.com - Accessed 23 Aug. 2021.

[24] Source: Supplier for Assistep – https://liveeasyinc.com/products/assistep/ - Accessed 23 Aug. 2021.

[25] Source: Supplier for elevator – https://www.vacuumelevators.com - Accessed 23 Aug. 2021.

[26] Source: Supplier for stair lift – https://access.nsm-seating.com/midwest/stair-lifts/ - Accessed 23 Aug. 2021.

[27] Source: Supplier for assistive aids – https://www.wellwise.ca/en-ca/ - Accessed 23 Aug. 2021.

[28] Source: Modifying your bathtub – https://imperialbath.net - Accessed 23 Aug. 2021.

[29] Source: Laundry soap strips, etc. (no plastic) https://www.tru.earth - Accessed 23 Aug. 2021.

[30] Source: Grab bars – all styles - https://www.healthcraftproducts.com/products/bathroom-safety/?gclid=EAIaIQobChMIrJzB5M6S8gIVApezCh0VegXiEAAYASAAEgILHPD_BwE - Accessed 23 Aug. 2021.

[31] Retirement home options: (1) Independent living, (2) Semi-assisted living, (3) Assisted living

[32] Source: CMHC financing options – https://www.cmhc-schl.gc.ca/en/consumers/owning-a-home/aging-in-place/mortgage-financing-options-for-people-55-and-above - Accessed 23 Aug. 2021.

[33] Source: Housing co-operative – https://settlement.org/ontario/housing/living-in-ontario/housing-basics/what-is-a-housing-co-operative/ - Accessed 23 Aug. 2021.

[34] Source: Housing options for seniors – https://www.senioradvisor.com/blog/2015/09/canadas-supportive-housing-options-for-seniors/ - Accessed 23 Aug. 2021.

[35] Source: Seniors housing guide – https://www.aplaceformom.com/planning-and-advice/articles/canada-seniors-housing-guide - Accessed 23 Aug. 2021.

[36] Platinum Rule: "Do unto others as *they* would want done to *them.*"

[37] Source: Background check – https://nationalpardon.org/free-background-check-canada/ - Accessed 23 Aug. 2021.

[38] Source: Ageing in place – https://www.rehabmagazine.ca/health-care/aging-in-place-myth-or-reality/ –https://www.apa.org/pi/aging/resources/guides/myth-reality.pdf - Accessed 23 Aug. 2021.

[39] Source: Kaizen - https://www.investopedia.com/terms/k/kaizen.asp - Accessed 23 Aug. 2021.

[40] Source: Speech-Language & Audiology Canada – https://www.sac-oac.ca/seniors - Accessed 23 Aug. 2021.

[41] Source: No salt cooking herbs – https://mrsdash.com - Accessed 23 Aug. 2021.

[42] Source: Senior's top Fears of Aging - https://info.daystarseattle.com/senior-living-blog/understanding-your-aging-parents-seniors-top-10-fears

[43] Source: Advance care planning – https://www.dying-withdignity.ca/download_your_advance_care_planning_kit?utm_campaign=webinar_acp_clancy_recording_b&utm_medium=email&utm_source=dwdcanada - Accessed 23 Aug. 2021.

[44] Source: Advance care planning – https://www.dyingwith-dignity.ca/acp_videos?utm_campaign=webinar_acp_clancy_recording_b&utm_medium=email&utm_source=dwdcanada - Accessed 23 Aug. 2021.

[45] Source: Executor Help – How to settle an estate – https://www.davidedey.com - Accessed 23 Aug. 2021.

[46] Source: Senior independence article – https://www.nextavenue.org/safety-priority-independence-older-parents/ - Accessed 23 Aug. 2021.

[47] Source: Difficult conversations – https://www.nextavenue.org/have-difficult-conversations-with-your-aging-parents/ - Accessed 23 Aug. 2021.

[48] Please include all aspects of your life – Geographical, Physical, Emotional, and Psychological well-being.

CPSIA information can be obtained
at www.ICGtesting.com
Printed in the USA
LVHW031032251122
733960LV00002B/375

9 781039 128880